Back and Neck Health

MAYO CLINIC PRESS

MAYO CLINIC

Medical Editor
Mohamad Bydon, M.D.

Editorial Director
Paula M. Marlow Limbeck

Senior Editor
Karen R. Wallevand

Senior Product Manager
Daniel J. Harke

Art Director
Stewart J. Koski

Illustration, Photography and Production
Benjamin (Ben) J. Hanson, Joanna R. King, Michael A. King, Kent McDaniel, Matthew C. Meyer

Editorial Research Librarians
Abbie Y. Brown, Edward (Eddy) S. Morrow Jr., Erika A. Riggin, Katherine (Katie) J. Warner

Copy Editors
Miranda M. Attlesey, Alison K. Baker, Nancy J. Jacoby, Julie M. Maas

Indexer
Carol Roberts

Administrative Assistant
Terri L. Zanto Strausbauch

Contributors
J.D. Bartleson, M.D., Jeffrey S. Brault, D.O., Kari A. Cornell, Christine (Christy) L. Hunt, D.O., Jason S. Eldrige, M.D., Kristin L. Garlanger, D.O., Kingsley Adobe-Iyamah, M.D., Mark A. Jensen, P.T., Timothy J. Kaufmann, M.D., William E. Krauss, M.D., Heather L. LaBruna, Mark K. Lyons, M.D., W. Richard Marsh, M.D., Bradly (Brad) W. Prigge, Randy A. Shelerud, M.D., Laura M. Waxman, Jodi Cooper-Wentz

Published by Mayo Clinic Press

For bulk sales to employers, member groups and health-related companies, contact Mayo Clinic, 200 First St. SW, Rochester, MN 55905, call 800-430-9699, or send an email to SpecialSalesMayoBooks@mayo.edu.

ISBN 978-1-893005-63-1

Library of Congress Control Number: 2020938350

Printed in the United States of America

Contents

Preface

As a neurosurgeon specializing in spinal surgery, I see patients every day whose lives are deeply impacted by back and neck pain, and I understand how frustrating and debilitating back and neck conditions can be. We're all busy and active, and back and neck health is important to all of us.

As you'll learn from this book, back and neck pain are among the top reasons people see their primary care doctors. Statistics show that approximately 80% of us will experience at least one significant episode of back pain at some point in our lives. Many of us will also experience neck pain.

If you're one of many people living with a back or neck condition, you understand the impact on your life and that of your family. You know how hard it can be to do those things that you enjoy or to accomplish what used to be simple activities. You may also have found that getting reliable information on your condition can be a challenge.

This book, written by Mayo Clinic authorities on back and neck health, is meant to provide you with comprehensive and up-to-date information on your back or neck condition, along with recommendations on when to seek medical care and guidance.

Whether you're dealing with back or neck pain for the first time or you've been living with your condition for years, in the pages that follow, you'll find helpful information on the underlying causes of back and neck conditions, why you feel pain and, most importantly, how best to treat your problem.

Many of my patients come to me expecting that they'll need surgery to treat their conditions. In some cases, surgery is necessary and is the best solution to the problem. However, surgery isn't always the answer. There are other treatments that can effectively treat back and neck pain.

My hope is that by gaining a better understanding of common back and neck problems and being equipped with the latest information on how to treat them, you can make informed decisions about your care so that you can successfully manage your condition and enjoy an improved quality of life.

It has been my pleasure to help create *Back and Neck Health*, and I am grateful for the contributions of my colleagues.

Mohamad Bydon, M.D.

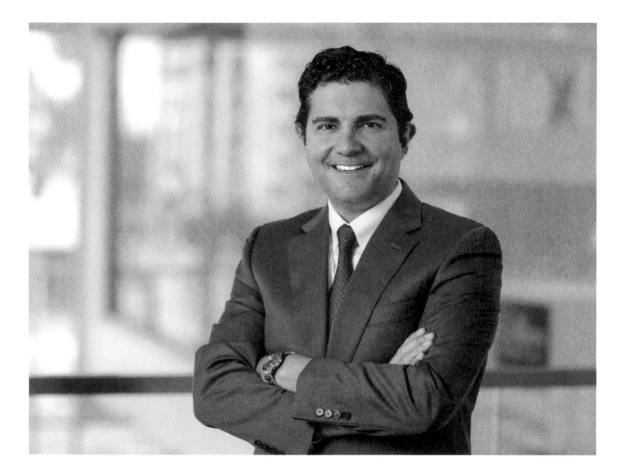

Mohamad Bydon, M.D., is a professor of neurosurgery, orthopedic surgery and health services research at Mayo Clinic in Rochester, Minn. As a neurosurgeon, he specializes in complex spine surgery, spinal oncology and minimally invasive spine surgery. Dr. Bydon is a graduate of Dartmouth College and Yale University School of Medicine. He completed his medical residency and a clinical fellowship at Johns Hopkins Hospital. At Mayo Clinic, Dr. Bydon see patients regularly and has received honors for his exceptional delivery of patient care. He also serves as assistant dean of education at Mayo Clinic College of Medicine and Science and medical director of the Mayo Clinic Enterprise Registry, a real-time patient safety and outcomes platform that integrates data from Mayo Clinic's hospitals and clinics nationwide. In addition, Dr. Bydon is the principal investigator of the Mayo Clinic Neuro-Informatics Laboratory, dedicated to advancing neurological patient care and safety. Dr. Bydon is a frequent lecturer and has authored more than 250 peer-reviewed manuscripts and hundreds of book chapters, abstracts and other publications. He is currently editor-in-chief of the *International Journal of Neuroscience* and holds reviewer responsibilities for several other scientific publications.

Introduction

Back pain can stop you in your tracks. Whether you're moving, sitting or lying still, all you know is that your back hurts, and the pain consumes you. It's hard to concentrate, it's hard to do things and it's virtually impossible to ignore the pain.

When back pain strikes, your normal routine is interrupted. You may find it difficult to go to work, especially if your job involves physical labor or standing or sitting at a desk all day. Things you enjoy outside of work, perhaps going for a walk, playing a round of golf, or taking part in activities with your children or grandchildren, quickly become off-limits. You may find it's even painful to laugh or carry on a conversation.

Unfortunately, it's easy for the situation to spin out of control. Because it hurts when you move, you don't move, you don't do things. As a result, your body becomes de-conditioned, heightening the pain and making you even more frightened to be active. Before long, simply sitting around and doing nothing leaves you feeling exhausted.

Neck pain isn't a whole lot better. Like back pain, it can consume your life and sideline your daily routine. When it hurts to move your neck, it becomes easier to do nothing. You don't go to the gym, you turn down a trip to the ballgame with friends, you let the weeds overtake your garden.

All you want to is feel better, but you're beginning to wonder if you'll ever be your old self again.

YOU'RE NOT ALONE

Back and neck pain are common complaints. When you think of all of the work that your back and neck do each day — constantly moving, bending and twisting as you go about your day-to-day activities — it's not surprising that problems develop. A misstep or a wrong move and the mechanical actions of your spine can get out of sync, causing injury and pain. A muscle may pull, a ligament tear, a bone fracture or a nerve become pinched.

It's estimated that more than 80% of American adults will experience at least one bout of back pain during their lifetimes. Back injury is the most common cause of job-related disability and a leading contributor to missed days of work. A survey of U.S. workers found that about 1 in 4 has experienced low back pain at some point in his or her life.

Back pain has few boundaries. Men and women of all backgrounds are affected. The older you are, the more likely your chance of encountering a bout of back pain. Prevalence of low back pain increases with age, with the highest incidence occurring in individuals in their 50s and 60s.

But back injury isn't limited to middle-aged and older individuals. In recent years, doctors have begun to see more teens and young adults with low back pain. Speculation has it that this may be partly due to more young people hunching over laptop computers, tablets and other electronic devices.

Neck pain, while less frequent, also is a common complaint. Studies suggest that somewhere between 10% and 30% of the adult population is bothered by neck pain. Similar to back pain, it peaks in middle age. However, unlike back pain, neck pain tends to be more common in women than in men.

Most often, an episode of back or neck pain is a short-term event that resolves over a period of days or weeks. You stretch or twist something and feel the pain for a period of time, and then it gradually gets better. But not everyone is that fortunate.

For some people, the pain continues beyond the normal period of healing, lasting months or even years. In other individuals, the pain improves for a period of time but recurs. And each time it recurs, the longer it seems to last.

MANY CAUSES

Back and neck pain can develop for a variety of reasons. Typically, the pain is associated with some type of mechanical damage — a pull or a tear, a slip or a crack, a pinch or a bulge. It may be something seemingly trivial that triggered the event, such as bending over, sneezing or coughing. Or it may be something more serious, such as an accident or a traumatic injury.

Because back and neck pain are so common, you may think they're inevitable. However, certain factors and occupations put you at greater risk. Your odds of experiencing back pain are increased if you smoke, are overweight, are inactive, or are experiencing stress, anxiety or depression.

A physically demanding job, especially one involving heavy lifting, unbalanced stretching or bending, or subtle, repeated actions, can increase your risk. So can a sedentary job sitting at a desk or in front of a computer all day. A sudden change in activity also can be a problem, for instance, not getting any exercise during the week and then diving into a strenuous weekend workout.

Finally, and not surprisingly, age and years of wear and tear on your bones, muscles and ligaments put you at increased risk. Back and neck pain associated with wear and tear (degeneration) often tends to develop more gradually.

And it may be that pain isn't your only concern. It's not uncommon for back and neck pain to be accompanied by other symptoms, such as weakness, numbness and difficulty with certain movements. And the pain may spread. Back pain may extend down one or both legs. Neck pain can migrate to your shoulders and arms.

Your back or neck may be the culprit, but much of your body may be feeling it.

A WEIGHTY TOLL

When your pain first developed, you may not have thought too much about it. You figured in a day or two it would be gone. But as the problem persisted and it started to limit your daily activities, you began to get worried. What does the pain mean? How long will it last? Should I see a doctor?

Should I go to work? Can I afford to miss work?

Back and neck pain can take a big toll on your life. Fear and worry, along with difficulty sleeping, can leave you feeling irritable. In addition, you may feel guilty about not being able to participate in events or activities or having to hand off some of your daily tasks to family members, friends or co-workers.

If you're not careful, a vicious cycle can develop. The more stressed you become, the more pain you experience. The greater the pain, the greater the stress, and so on. This cycle can be difficult to break. For some people, it can lead to depression.

Beyond the emotional toll are the financial costs of back and neck pain. First, there are the direct costs to you for time spent at the doctor, missed days of work, and medicines and other treatments you may have tried. Then there are the societal costs. Taking into account both the actual costs of treatment for back and neck pain as well as the associated costs to employers in missed days of work, loss of employee productivity and disability benefits, the price tag is estimated well into the *billions* of dollars.

An analysis of health care spending in the United States published in 2020 by the *Journal of the American Medical Association* found that in recent years, treatment of low back pain and neck pain accounted for the highest amounts of spending by both private and public insurers.

GETTING YOUR LIFE BACK

So, what are we saying? If you have back or neck pain you're doomed? Far from it!

Clearly, the two are common, and they're costly. But these are conditions that can be successfully treated. If you've lived with back or neck pain for a long time, or you know of someone who has, don't feel that there's nothing that can be done.

Doctors and researchers continue to explore new therapies for the treatment of back and neck pain, as well as refine existing ones. Most often, back and neck pain can be treated without surgery. Sometimes, basic measures such as rest, exercise, and ice and heat are the answer. Other times, more-specific interventions such as physical therapy, injections or medication can help resolve the pain. Surgery is reserved for those instances in which conservative measures don't bring any improvements and there's evidence that surgery can relieve your symptoms.

This process can take time. It may take a while to identify the source of your pain, and it's not always possible to find a specific source. In addition, your doctor may need to experiment with a couple of different treatment approaches before he or she finds the one that works. Though it can be difficult, having a little patience helps.

In the chapters that follow, we discuss different types of back and neck pain, and what can cause them. As you will find out, many conditions can produce pain. That's why figuring out the source of your pain can take time. You'll also learn the different ways to treat back and neck pain. This includes steps you can take on your own at home, several interventional approaches and different types of surgery. The final chapter of the book focuses on lifestyle. It offers advice on what you can do to keep your back and neck healthy and prevent previous problems from recurring.

It's our hope and intent that a complete understanding of the causes and treatment of back and neck pain can help you find the pain relief you seek.

Understanding your back and neck

Your spine

The human spine is an amazing structure, and one of the most important parts of your body. Your spine runs from the base of your skull down the length of your back, extending all the way to your pelvis. Also known as your backbone, your spine is what gives your body structure and support. Without it, you couldn't keep yourself upright or move!

You might picture your spine as similar to a ladder or scaffold. It provides a central framework for your body's skeletal system and all of its components, including your muscular and nervous systems. No matter what you're doing — whether you're standing, sitting, bending, twisting or lifting — your spine is always at work, supporting your body.

To help you understand why your back or neck is hurting, it helps to know more about your spine, how it works and its key functions. First of all, your spine is a protector. It provides a bony barrier, safeguarding your spinal cord and nerves. Your spine also serves as your body's structural powerhouse, supporting your body weight and the transfer of weight from one part of your body to another as you move. And your spine is a facilitator, providing the mechanism that makes it possible for your body to flex, extend, twist, and turn to the left and right.

To accomplish these critical functions, all of the components that make up your spine must work together and efficiently. When something goes wrong, problems can develop. And a problem with your spine may affect other areas of your body — even areas that seem completely unrelated. For example, pain or numbness in a leg may be traced to a pinched nerve in your lower back.

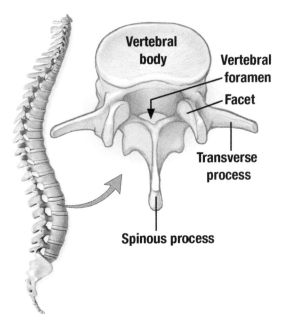

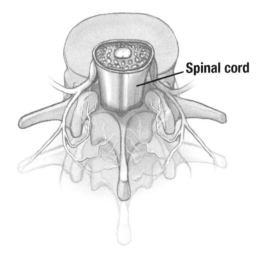

Vertebral body

Vertebral foramen

Facet

Transverse process

Spinous process

Spinal cord

Vertebrae. The spine is composed of 33 small interlocking bones called vertebrae. Each bone (vertebra) contains delicate structures that allow the bones to stack on top of one another and muscles to attach to them.

Spinal cord. In the center of each vertebra is a small hole called the vertebral foramen that forms the spinal canal. The spinal canal houses the spinal cord and spinal nerves, which extend from the base of the brain to the pelvis.

A brief review of your spinal anatomy will help you understand how your spine functions and some of the problems that can develop due to natural aging or injury.

VERTEBRAE

Your spine is made up of 33 spool-shaped bones collectively known as vertebrae. An individual bone is called a vertebra. Each vertebra is about an inch thick and stacked one on top of another. The vertebrae are supported by ligaments and connected to muscles that extend throughout the body.

Each vertebra that forms your spine consists of the following parts:

- **Vertebral body.** The vertebral body is the somewhat thick, flat main part of the bone that bears the most weight. The vertebral body stacks on top of the vertebra below it and is the foundation for the vertebra above it.
- **Vertebral foramen.** The vertebral foramen is the triangular shaped hole that contains the spinal cord and nerves. One vertebral foramen located on top of another forms the spinal canal. One of the most important functions of the spine is protecting the spinal cord.

- **Spinous process.** The spinous process is the bony protrusion on the back of each vertebra. This protrusion is what you feel when you run your hand down the middle of your neck and back.
- **Transverse process.** On each side of a vertebra is a bony protrusion called the transverse process. Muscles and ligaments attach to and connect the vertebrae at these processes.
- **Facet.** On each side of a vertebra is an area where one vertebra connects to another. The connection points between the vertebrae are referred to as the facet joints.

Spinal regions

The spine's vertebrae are broken down into four distinct regions.

Cervical spine The cervical spine is delicate and includes the seven vertebrae that make up the neck. The first cervical vertebra is called the atlas, and it secures your head to your neck. This is where the neck has the greatest flexibility and extension, making it possible for you to do things such as nod your head yes. The second vertebra is the axis. It primarily allows your neck to rotate, as when you shake your head no. The third through the seventh vertebrae can extend and rotate to a lesser degree, as well as bend to the side. They help make it possible for you to touch your ear to your shoulder, for example. Of the four spinal regions, the cervical spine has the greatest range of motion.

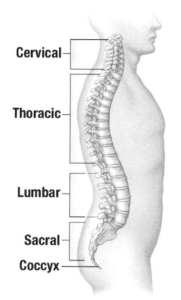

Spinal regions. The spine is divided into four main regions: cervical, thoracic, lumbar and sacral. Each region has specific characteristics and functions. At the base of the spine is the coccyx, also known as the tailbone.

Thoracic spine The thoracic spine consists of the 12 bones of the middle back and rib area. Each of the thoracic vertebrae connect to your rib bones, providing support to the rib cage, which houses and protects your lungs and heart. Because the thoracic region connects to your ribs, it is the least mobile part of your back.

Lumbar spine Also known as the lower back area, the lumber spine is made up of five bones, which carry most of your body's weight. The lumbar spine isn't as mobile as the cervical spine, but it does have a greater range of motion than the thoracic spine.

Sacrum and coccyx The vertebrae at the bottom of your spine include the sacrum and the coccyx, also known as the tailbone. The sacrum consists of five fused vertebrae that form a large bone shaped like a wedge. The sacrum helps transfer weight from your spine to your pelvis, the heart-shaped bone that anchors your hip bones and supports the base of your spine. The coccyx is composed of the last four vertebrae of the lower spine. Like the sacrum, these bones are fused together.

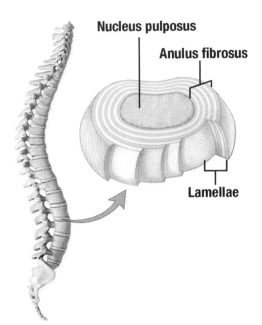

DISKS

Located between each of your vertebrae are disks, which serve as cushions and shock absorbers between the bones. Each disk is composed of a soft, gel-like interior (nucleus pulposus) that contains mostly water. This interior is surrounded by a harder, rubberlike outer coating. The outer coating is made of 10 to 20 sheets of tissue called lamellae. Lamellae consist of collagen, a connective tissue made of protein that gives bones, tendons and ligaments structure. Lamellae are firm and able to support heavy loads, but still flexible and bendable enough to allow movement.

In addition to separating your vertebrae, disks have other key functions. They transfer weight between the vertebrae, provide space between the bones to allow for movement, and cushion the vertebrae and spine as your body moves. Disks compress to absorb a weighted load and relax when the load is released.

Disk. A spinal disk has a soft, gel-like interior called the nucleus pulposus. The interior is encased by a tougher, rubbery exterior called the anulus fibrosis. The exterior is composed of sheets of tissue called lamellae.

Spinal disks account for about one-quarter of your spine's height. While they're located between each vertebra of the spine, they're not the same thickness. Disks are thinnest in the thoracic region, where vertebrae are more delicate, and thickest in the lumbar area, where the vertebrae are bigger and load bearing.

FACET JOINTS

Facet joints are the locations where one vertebra connects to the next. These joints help

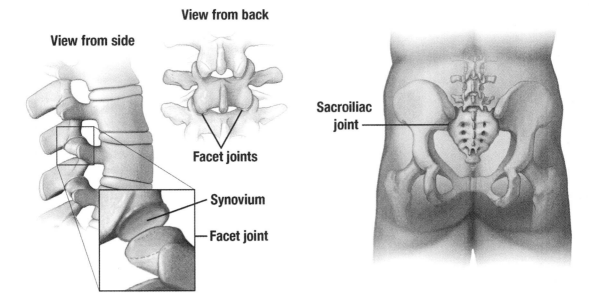

View from side

View from back

Facet joints

Synovium

Facet joint

Sacroiliac joint

Facet joint. Facet joints are the connection points between the bones of the vertebrae. These joints allow the spine to twist and bend while keeping your back from moving too far forward or twisting uncontrollably.

Sacroiliac joint. There are two sacroiliac joints. These large, strong joints connect the base of the spine (sacrum) to each side of the pelvis. Strong ligaments and muscles support the sacroiliac joints.

keep your spine aligned as it moves, and allow the spine to flex, extend and rotate. Similar to other joints in your body, facet joints contain a smooth membrane called synovium, which produces a fluid that lubricates the joints so they can glide and pivot. Most vertebral segments contain synovial facet joints on both the right and left sides.

lows less spinal motion. These are known as fibrocartilaginous joints. There are also two large joints, known as the sacroiliac joints, that connect the bottom portion of the spine (sacrum) and the upper pelvis. The sacroiliac joints act as shock absorbers, helping transfer weight and energy between your upper body and your legs.

Other joints

Other spinal joints are lined with flexible connective tissue called cartilage, which al-

NERVES

Your spine serves as the main passageway for your spinal cord and other nerves within

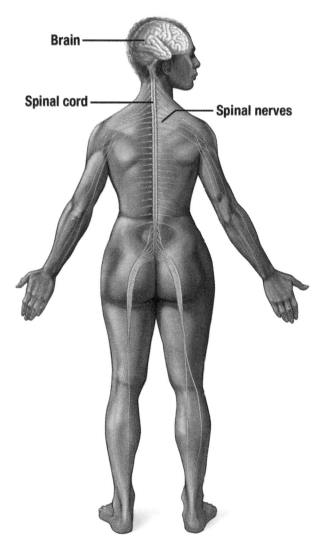

Brain

Spinal cord

Spinal nerves

Peripheral nerves. The peripheral nervous system is a network of pairs of motor and sensory nerves that connect the brain and spinal cord (central nervous system) to the entire human body. The peripheral nerves control body functions related to sensation, movement and motor coordination. Damage to any part of a nerve can create dysfunction within the peripheral nervous system.

your nervous system. The spinal cord is a ropelike column of nerves that links your brain to the nerves in your arms, legs and trunk. The spinal cord begins at the base of your brain and runs down the center of each vertebra (vertebral column), ending where your lumbar region begins. The spinal cord is made up of the same tissue found in the brain.

An astounding 31 pairs of nerves run through the center of your spine. Between each vertebra, two nerves exit the spinal column, one on each side. One of the nerves extends to the left side of your body, while the other feeds to your right side. These nerves branch out from your spine to adjacent muscles and tissues.

Your spinal nerves carry messages — including sensations of pain, injury, heat and cold detected within the tissues and muscles of your arms, legs and core body — to your brain. And they relay messages in the opposite direction, such as instructing your muscles to move. Within your muscles are what are called sensory cells that are designed to read nerve messages. Your muscles respond by lengthening or contracting as instructed.

If a spinal nerve is injured — if it becomes restricted or pinched — your brain may respond to the injury with messages that cause you to feel pain. An example is the sciatic nerve, a large collection of lumbar and sacral nerves that branches from your lower back, extends over the buttocks and travels down the back of your legs. When this nerve becomes pinched, pain may begin in the lower back and buttocks and radiate down a leg, sometimes even affecting your foot. If there's enough pressure on the nerve, your leg may become numb or the leg muscles may feel weak.

LIGAMENTS

Ligaments are tough, fibrous bands of tissue made up of the connective proteins elastin and collagen. Ligaments connect to spinal vertebrae and help hold the vertebrae in place.

In conjunction with your muscles, ligaments allow you to bend forward and backward, turn, twist, and lift. Your ligaments are a bit like rubber bands. They absorb excess movement and bring the movement under control, limiting how far your spine can move. This keeps your spine safe, helping to protect it from injury. The ligaments in your back and neck are also interwoven with many nerves. These nerves alert your brain to the position of your head and neck, helping to keep your spine stable.

Your spine is made up of a variety of ligaments. Two main ligaments — the anterior longitudinal ligament (ALL) and the posterior longitudinal ligament (PLL) — extend from the top of your spine to the bottom, but serve different purposes. The anterior longitudinal ligament prevents hyperextension of your spine, which happens when your spine is pushed too far backward, either at the neck or in the lower back. The

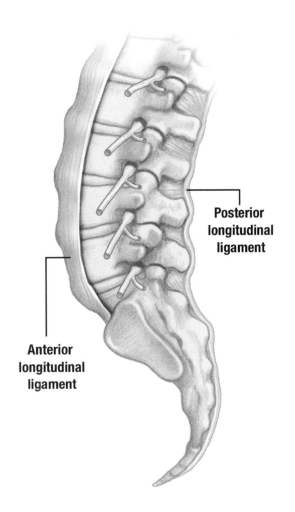

Posterior longitudinal ligament

Anterior longitudinal ligament

Ligaments. Ligaments are strong fibrous bands that hold vertebrae together, stabilize the spine and protect the disks. The spine contains a number of ligaments that help bind the spinal column. Two major ligaments that run the length of the spine are the anterior longitudinal ligament (ALL) and the posterior longitudinal ligament (PLL). These ligaments strengthen spinal disks to help prevent the disks from rupturing (disk herniation).

posterior longitudinal ligament prevents hyperflexion of your neck or lower back. This occurs when the spine is flexed too far forward.

TENDONS

Tendons are fibrous cords of tissue that attach the muscles in your back and abdomen to your spine and allow for movement. The tendons in your back tend to be shorter than those in other parts of your body, and they work a bit differently. The intricate system of internal tendons that attach to your back muscles generates added strength, power and tension in the muscles. This is important because of all of the strain, including from heavy lifting, placed on your back muscles.

MUSCLES

Many layers of muscles, both long and short, extend across your neck and back. Some of the muscles (intrinsic muscles) connect vertebrae in your spine to one another. Other muscles (extrinsic muscles) link your spine to other parts of your body, such as your head, arms and legs.

Unlike the muscles located in your arms or legs that attach to bone in one location, your back and spinal muscles tend to fan out and usually attach to more than one bone. These muscles work together, supporting your weight and allowing your body to move. Each muscle has a specific job.

Intrinsic muscles

Intrinsic muscles attach vertebrae to one another or to your skull. These muscles, which facilitate movement and maintain posture, are surrounded by fibrous connective tissue called deep fascia. Intrinsic muscles fall into three groups — superficial, intermediate and deep. The superficial muscles lie closest to the surface of your back. Intermediate muscles are located between the superficial and deep muscles. Deep muscles, as their names suggests, are the deepest.

Superficial muscles The superficial muscles include the splenius capitis muscle. It connects your lowest cervical vertebra with the top four thoracic vertebrae and the ligament that extends down the back of your neck (ligamentum nuchae). Another superficial muscle, the cervicis muscle, also connects vertebrae in your neck with your thoracic vertebrae. The splenius capitis and the cervicis muscles work together so that you can move your head and neck to the left and right.

Intermediate muscles The erector spinae muscles are three columns of muscles that overlap one another. The same ligament attaches all three of these muscle columns to the lumbar vertebrae, the sacrum and the sacroiliac ligaments. The sacroiliac ligament runs behind the pelvis and connects the sacrum to the top of the pelvis.

Deep muscles A deep layer of intrinsic muscles helps make it possible to extend your head and neck, stabilizes your vertebrae,

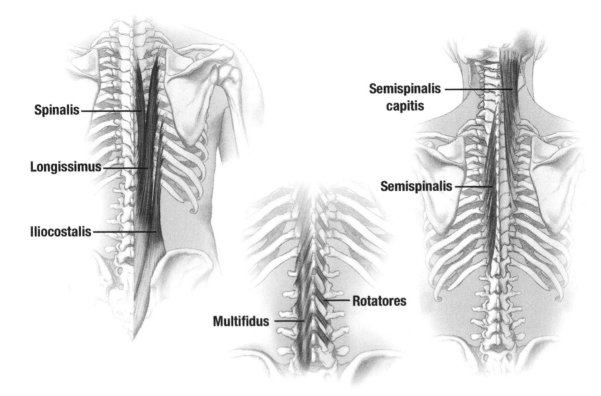

Intrinsic muscles. The deep intrinsic muscles of the back and neck extend from the base of the skull to the pelvis. These are short, well-developed muscles that fuse with spinal vertebrae. Deep muscles help stabilize the spine as well as allow the spine to bend and twist.

and allows the vertebrae to rotate. These deep muscles include the semispinalis, multifidus and rotatores muscles.

Extrinsic muscles

Extrinsic muscles extend beyond your back, attaching the vertebrae of the spine to your arms, legs, shoulders, pelvis and ribs. These muscles fall into two categories — superficial muscles and intermediate muscles.

Superficial extrinsic muscles, such as the trapezius and latissimus dorsi muscles, help make it possible for you to move your shoulders, neck, arms and upper trunk.

Intermediate extrinsic muscles stretch from your spine to your ribs and are located below the superficial muscles. Intermediate muscles include the superior and inferior serratus posterior, which are involved in breathing and help your rib cage expand and contract.

Upper back and neck Extrinsic muscles located in the upper back and neck include the following:

- **Latissimus dorsi.** It serves as the main extrinsic muscle, connecting six of your thoracic vertebrae to your armpit (axilla). This muscle lifts and lowers the trunk of your body.
- **Trapezius.** The trapezius fans out across your shoulder, attaching the lowest cervical vertebra and several thoracic vertebrae to your shoulder blade (scapula). The muscle helps you to tilt and turn your head and neck, shrug your shoulders, and twist your arms.
- **Rhomboids.** The rhomboids also connect the lowest cervical vertebra and a few thoracic vertebrae with your scapula. Like the trapezius, these muscles help move your shoulders.
- **Serratus posterior.** It has two parts, the superior and the inferior. The superior is located between your neck and the top of your rib cage and it connects the lowest cervical vertebra and the first three thoracic vertebrae with your ribs. This muscle helps to lift your ribs. The inferior connects the lower thoracic vertebrae with your first two lumber vertebrae. This muscle helps to lowers your ribs.

Lower back and pelvis Extrinsic muscles in your lower back and abdomen connect the lumbar vertebrae to your pelvis. These muscles help you to move your hips and legs. Hip motion allows your lumbar spine to bend, extend or lift heavy loads.

- **Quadratus lumborum.** The deepest abdominal muscle, this muscle helps to stabilize your spine and allows you to move your lower back from left to right. The rectangular-shaped muscle links your bottom rib with the sides of your first four lumbar vertebrae and the top of your pelvis.
- **Psoas major.** The psoas major muscle, a long muscle in the lower back, works with the muscle that links the top of your pelvis with the top of your femur (iliacus) so that you can flex your lower trunk and your thigh.
- **Hip (extensors), glutes and hamstrings.** When you bend forward, your hip muscles, glutes, and hamstring muscles are activated.
- **Pelvic.** Your pelvic muscles play a key role in the shifting of weight from the legs to the pelvis and then up the spine.

Core muscles

Your abdominal (core) muscles also are important to back health. These muscles include the transversus abdominis, rectus abdominis, and the internal and external oblique muscles. Your core muscles work with your back muscles to help keep your spine aligned, as well as allow you to bend forward at your lower back and turn from side to side.

Strong and balanced core muscles are important to good posture, ease of movement and your ability to lift heavy objects.

- **Transversus abdominis.** It's the deepest core muscle, attaching to your lumbar vertebrae through a layer of fascia. This

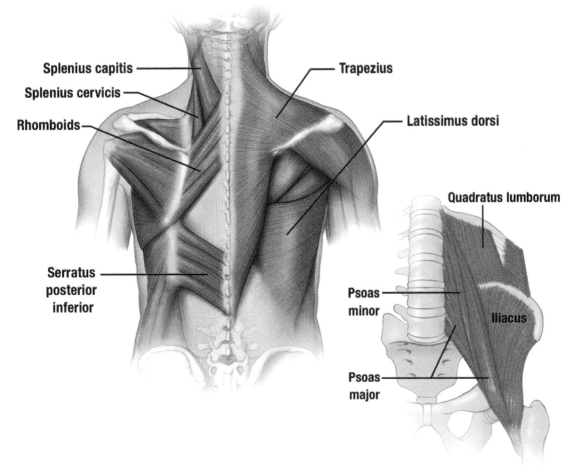

Splenius capitis

Splenius cervicis

Rhomboids

Trapezius

Latissimus dorsi

Quadratus lumborum

Serratus
posterior
inferior

Psoas
minor

Iliacus

Psoas
major

Extrinsic muscles. The superficial extrinsic muscles of the neck and back are located on top of the intermediate extrinsic muscles and are covered by layers of fat, tissue and skin. Extrinsic muscles provide for movement of the shoulders and upper body and assist with breathing (respiration).

---

key muscle provides overall support to your spine.

- **Internal and external obliques.** These muscles are layered on top of the transversus abdominis. They help control spinal rotation.
- **Rectus abdominis.** It extends from the bottom of your rib cage to the top of your pubic bone, helping you to bend your lower back and trunk.

YOUR SPINE IN ACTION

Your spine is engineered for movement. Each time you take a step, turn or twist, nerve cells in your muscles send messages along nerve pathways to your spinal cord and up to your brain. These messages provide instructions that your brain communicates to the rest of your body, indicating what action your body needs to take.

In response to the messages they receive, your muscles, ligaments, tendons and other tissues work together either to lengthen and stretch or to tighten and contract, making it possible for you to move. When all the coordinating parts of your spine are healthy, fully functioning and working together, you're able perform most any task easily and without pain.

But when something goes wrong, the whole system can be thrown out of whack. There are many ways that you might offset the natural movement of your spine and its components, injuring your back or neck in the process. For example, if you lift too heavy a load, you can strain a muscle. If you stretch too far when reaching for something, you can pull a ligament or tendon. If you bend the wrong way, you may pinch a nerve.

Beyond your back

It's also important to remember that the health of your spine affects more than your back and neck. It's integral to the functioning of your arms and legs.

Peripheral nerves are the nerves that branch out from the center of your spine, beginning at the neck and shoulders and extending to the tailbone. Among their other duties, these nerves control feeling and movement in your arms and legs.

The interconnectedness of your spinal nerves and peripheral nerves explains why pain you may first experience in your lower back may spread to one or both legs or feet. Or why pain that develops in your neck may extend to your arms or hands. Pain sensations are able to travel along this delicate but vast network of nerves.

AGE AND YOUR SPINE

With age, your spine naturally changes. During everyday use, it becomes less limber and flexible, part of a process called spinal degeneration. Over time, the rubbery disks that cushion the vertebrae dry out and lose some of the gel-like substance within their centers. With less gel, the disks become more rigid. They aren't able to cushion the bones of your back and neck as effectively as they once did, or provide needed support when you lift something heavy.

As disks lose their flexibility, they're more likely to tear or rupture. In addition, as the disks flatten, the vertebrae come closer together. In some cases, this can cause bone to rub against bone, leading to further degeneration.

Other parts of your spine change over time as well. Your ligaments may thicken and stiffen, reducing their ability to stretch. Facet joints can degrade due to wear and tear,

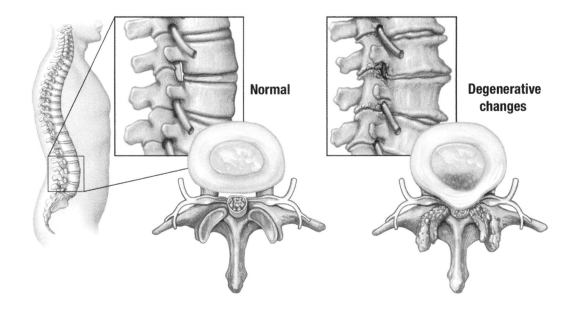

Spinal degeneration. Time, age, and wear and tear can damage the structures of the spine. Degenerative disease can affect all parts of the spine including vertebrae, disks and joints. Arthritis is a common type of degenerative disease.

making them less supportive. Vertebrae tend to remain reliably strong for about 50 years, but beyond age 50, bone density often decreases. Loss of density means your bones become weaker, increasing your risk of spinal fractures or bone malformations.

In addition, over time, the natural curve at the base of your neck (cervical lordosis) and the natural curve at the base of your spine (lumbar lordosis) gradually straighten out. These natural curves help your spine absorb shock, align your head with your pelvis and support the weight of your upper body. Without these curves, your spine is less adaptive when moving or when lifting or bending with heavy loads.

Changes such as these can lead to pain. If you're in pain, you may walk or move differently from normal. This can produce a domino effect called degenerative cascade, gradual but consistent wear and tear on key parts of the spine, including the disks, facet joints, ligaments and even the vertebrae themselves. When this occurs, your chance of injury increases.

In the next chapter, we talk more specifically about what causes back and neck pain and the different types of pain. You'll also read about factors that may place you at increased risk of back and neck injury.

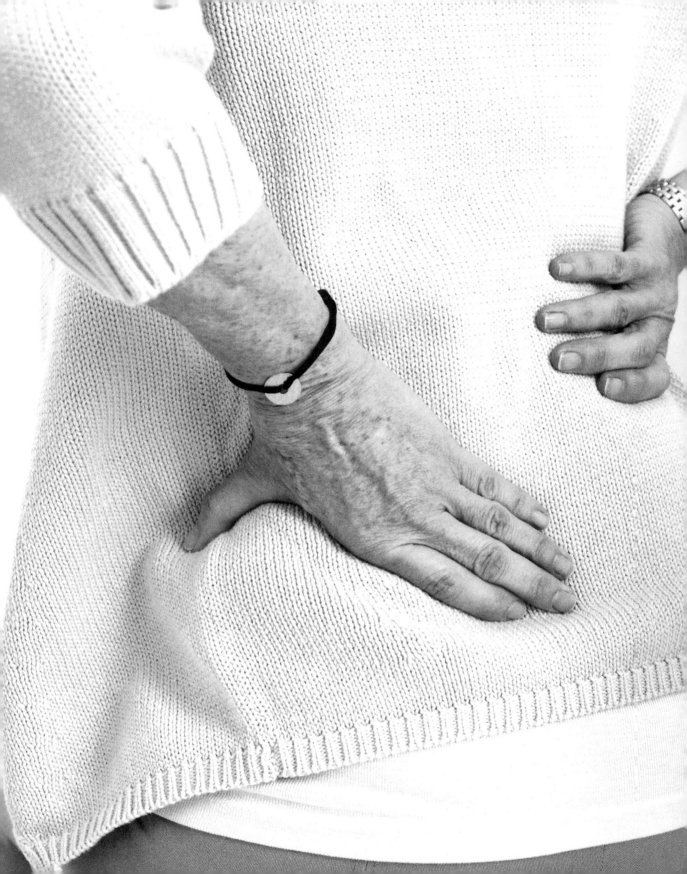

CHAPTER 2

Back and neck pain

Your back is killing you, and you have no idea why. Or perhaps it's your neck that's causing all of your troubles. What you do know is that what started out as a minor ache has developed into full-blown pain that bothers you day and night. What's worse, nothing you do seems to make it feel any better. Now you're not just in pain, you're frustrated.

In your quest for relief, it helps to know a bit more about factors that put you at increased risk of back and neck problems, and the different ways that pain may present itself.

WHAT PUTS YOU AT RISK?

Back and neck problems are common. Most people deal with at least one episode of back or neck pain at some point in their lives. As mentioned earlier, low back and neck pain are among the most common reasons why adults see a doctor, and back injury is the most common cause of job-related disability.

The age at which you start experiencing back or neck pain and how often you're bothered by such problems often has to do with your lifestyle, your occupation and your general health.

The good news is that you have some control over all of these things, with one exception — age.

Age

With age, the bones, joints, ligaments and disks of your back and neck naturally begin to show wear and tear. Ligaments stiffen and become less flexible. Disks dry out and become more rigid, causing them to burst or tear. Bones can lose their strength and become more vulnerable to fracture.

The wearing down of structures in your back and neck is called spinal degeneration, and it happens to all of us. As these structures weaken, they provide less support, increasing your risk of an injury.

Inactivity

Back pain is more common among people who aren't physically fit. If you don't exercise regularly and maintain some level of fitness, your risk of neck and back problems increases. Weekend warriors — people who exercise heavily on the weekends after being inactive all week — also are at greater risk of back and neck injury.

Regular exercise is very important because it strengthens the muscles, joints and bones that help support your back and neck. When you don't get enough exercise, your body's core muscles lose their strength and they don't provide adequate support to your spine.

Overweight

Carrying around additional weight places increased stress on your spine, straining joints and ligaments in the process. In addition, people who are overweight often don't get enough daily exercise to maintain core muscle strength, important to a healthy spine. Individuals who are overweight also tend to be at increased risk of diseases such as diabetes and osteoarthritis, which can increase your risk of back and neck problems.

Occupation

Any job, such as a construction worker or freight handler, that requires repetitive bending, lifting, pushing or pulling — particularly when it involves twisting or vibrating the spine — increases the risk of back and neck injury. A job that requires long hours sitting or standing without a break also puts you at greater risk of developing a back or neck condition.

Poor posture

Sitting or maintaining one position for too long isn't good for your back or your neck, especially if your posture is poor. Office jobs that involve long hours hunched over a computer can lead to back and neck pain, so can factory jobs in which you stand in one position for hours on end.

Poor posture, especially when combined with inactivity, puts stress on your spine and weakens muscles designed to support your neck and back. Neck muscles can also become strained when you hold your head in the same position for a long time, such as when staring at a computer or cradling a phone between your ear and shoulder.

Even reading in bed or grinding your teeth at night can lead to neck pain.

Stress and anxiety

When you're stressed, you may inadvertently tense up and strain the muscles in your neck and back. This can cause stiffness, soreness and pain. The more stressed you feel, the tighter your muscles become. If you're muscles are constantly tensed, you may also experience muscle spasms.

It's easy for a vicious cycle to develop. The more stressed you are, the greater your pain. The greater your pain, the more your stress.

Anxiety and depression can influence back and neck pain in that they may cause you to focus on the pain and increase your perception of its severity. In other words, the more you think about your pain, the worse it seems. It stands to reason, then, that if you've been diagnosed with an anxiety disorder or depression, treating those conditions may improve your pain and disability.

Smoking

So, what does smoking have to do with your back or neck? Smoking reduces blood flow to your lower spine, which can keep your body from delivering enough nutrients to the disks in your lower back. With inadequate nutrients, disks begin to dry out more quickly. Smoking has also been linked to increased bone resorption, reducing bone mass and increasing your risk of a fracture. Plus, if you do break a bone, smoking slows the healing process.

Osteoporosis

Individuals with osteoporosis are at increased risk of a spinal fracture. Osteoporosis causes bones to become weak and brittle — so brittle that a fall or even mild stresses such as bending over or coughing can fracture a bone in your back or neck.

Bone is living tissue that's constantly being broken down and replaced. Osteoporosis occurs when the creation of new bone doesn't keep pace with the loss of old bone. How likely you are to develop osteoporosis depends in part on how much bone mass you attained in your youth — most people reach their peak bone mass by age 30. The higher your peak bone mass, the more bone you have "in the bank" and the less likely you are to develop osteoporosis as you age.

Diabetes

Studies suggest diabetes can increase your risk of back and neck pain. Exactly how the two are interconnected is unknown at this point. It's possible diabetes may compromise blood vessels that supply the spine, resulting in reduced blood flow and increased spinal degeneration. More research is still needed, but in the meantime, good blood sugar control may be helpful in reducing tissue and bone degeneration of the spine.

UNDERSTANDING PAIN

Pain isn't something you should ignore. It's your body's way of telling you something is wrong. Pain can develop for many different reasons. It could be that you've experienced an injury. Or it may be a dysfunction in the way your nervous system is sending and receiving pain messages.

Pain also occurs in different degrees and dimensions. It may come on suddenly or develop slowly over time. You may feel a localized dull ache or you may have sharp, shooting pain that extends to your shoulder and arm or radiates down your leg. You may be in pain all of the time or experience pain only with certain movements.

Acute vs. chronic

There are two main categories of pain — acute and chronic. Acute pain is triggered by tissue or bone damage and is designed to protect you from further injury by alerting you that something is wrong. Chronic pain refers to persistent pain that continues after the injury has healed and that serves no real purpose.

Acute pain Acute pain is sudden pain that generally accompanies an illness, injury or surgery. The pain warns you that something is wrong so that you'll take steps to assess what's happening and prevent further injury. Acute pain is what you feel when you pull a muscle, break a bone or pinch a nerve.

Acute pain may last for a few minutes to a few hours or it can continue for days to a couple of weeks. Depending on the type of injury and its severity, the pain may range from mild to severe and it may present itself as sharp, stabbing, throbbing, stinging or shooting. Acute pain usually disappears with time and rest.

Subacute pain Sometimes, acute pain lasts longer than normal. If you continue to feel pain for more than a few weeks — beyond when it should normally begin to disappear — doctors will often refer to this as subacute pain. Subacute pain typically lasts between four and 12 weeks.

Chronic pain Chronic pain is another name for persistent pain — pain that continues beyond the time the injury or illness should have healed. Pain is generally categorized as chronic when it lasts 12 weeks or longer.

Chronic pain can occur for many reasons — the original injury doesn't heal properly, an infection isn't identified, a compressed nerve is left untreated, and so on. In most cases, though, chronic pain develops without any indication of an injury or illness. You begin to experience pain in your back or neck for no apparent reason and the pain doesn't go away.

As with acute pain, chronic pain spans the full range of sensations and intensities, from mild and achy to sharp and severe. Because the pain persists, chronic pain can be very frustrating and disruptive.

Chronic back pain and chronic neck pain are both common. And they're some of the most frequent reasons why people see a doctor.

Pain characteristics

Whether your pain comes on suddenly or it builds gradually, it can take many forms. Your pain may be a localized dull ache or a sharp and stabbing sensation that runs all the way down your leg. How your pain expresses itself can provide some clues as to a possible cause.

Localized vs. generalized Localized pain is limited to one area of your back or neck. Muscle-related pain resulting from tension, stress, overuse or a minor injury is usually localized. Generalized pain, meanwhile, refers to widespread pain. Generalized pain can cause your whole back to ache.

Radiating Radiating pain refers to pain that begins in one location and spreads. For

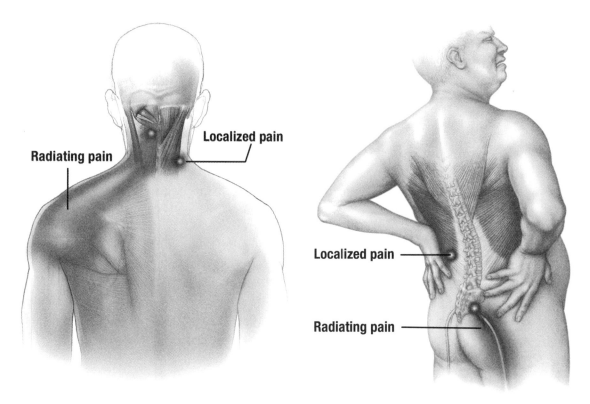

Pain. Common causes of muscle pain are tension, stress, overuse and minor injuries. This type of pain is usually localized, affecting a few muscles or a small part of your body. Radiating pain starts in one area and spreads until a larger area hurts. It's sometimes related to a nerve problem.

BEYOND THE PAIN

With many back and neck conditions you may experience more than just pain. Other signs and symptoms that may accompany your pain include:

- **Numbness and tingling.** These sensations occasionally go hand in hand with back and neck pain, especially when the pain radiates into an arm or leg. Numbness and tingling — also sometimes referred to as a "pins and needles" sensation — result when a nerve becomes pinched (compressed), irritated or damaged.
- **Loss of fine motor movement.** A compressed or irritated nerve can lead to weakness in the affected muscle. For example, as a muscle weakens it can become more difficult to pick up or hold on to things.
- **Difficulty walking.** Severe or prolonged pressure on spinal nerves can result in leg weakness and loss of feeling in the legs, causing difficulty walking.

example, the pain may begin in your neck and move to your shoulder and arm. Or it may originate in your lower back and extend to your buttocks and shoot down your leg.

Aching vs. stabbing vs. burning These terms are often used to describe how the pain feels. Aching pain is often, though not always, muscle related. In addition to the pain, muscles in the area where it hurts may be tender to the touch or feel tight and rigid.

Stabbing or burning pain, especially if the pain radiates, tends to be nerve related. This type of pain occurs when a nerve is pinched, damaged or irritated. With nerve-related pain, it might feel as if you're being jabbed with a sharp object or you may experience a prickling or tingling sensation.

Activity related With some back and neck conditions, the pain improves when you're inactive. Sitting or lying down relieves the pain. With other conditions, the opposite is true. You may find that you have less pain when you're walking or moving about than when you sit still.

You may also find that certain activities or movements trigger or worsen your pain. Simple things such as standing up, bending over, walking uphill, driving or lifting something may worsen your pain.

As you take steps to try to determine the cause of your back or neck condition, keep track of those things that seem to improve your pain, as well as activities or situations that make it worse. Choose activities that your neck and back tolerate best, and avoid those that make your symptoms worse.

WHEN TO SEE A DOCTOR

When you first experienced pain in your back or neck, you may have tried to treat the problem yourself to see if it would get better. In most cases, low back or neck pain improves significantly within three to six weeks. You may still have some pain for a longer period of time, but it's generally not severe and doesn't interfere with your daily activities. But how long should you wait for the pain to go away or your condition to get better?

Generally, it's recommended that you see a doctor if your symptoms don't start to get better within about three to four weeks. Also see a doctor if you begin to experience new or worsening symptoms, such as numbness, tingling or weakness in an arm or hand or leg or foot.

Are there times when you shouldn't wait — when you should see a doctor right away? Contact your doctor immediately if:
- Your pain follows a traumatic event, such as a fall or blow to your back
- Your pain is severe
- Your pain is accompanied by a fever of 100.4 F or higher

- You have loss of strength in a leg or arm
- You aren't able to control your bowels or bladder
- Your neck pain radiates down your arms or legs
- You have a headache, tingling or numbness along with neck pain

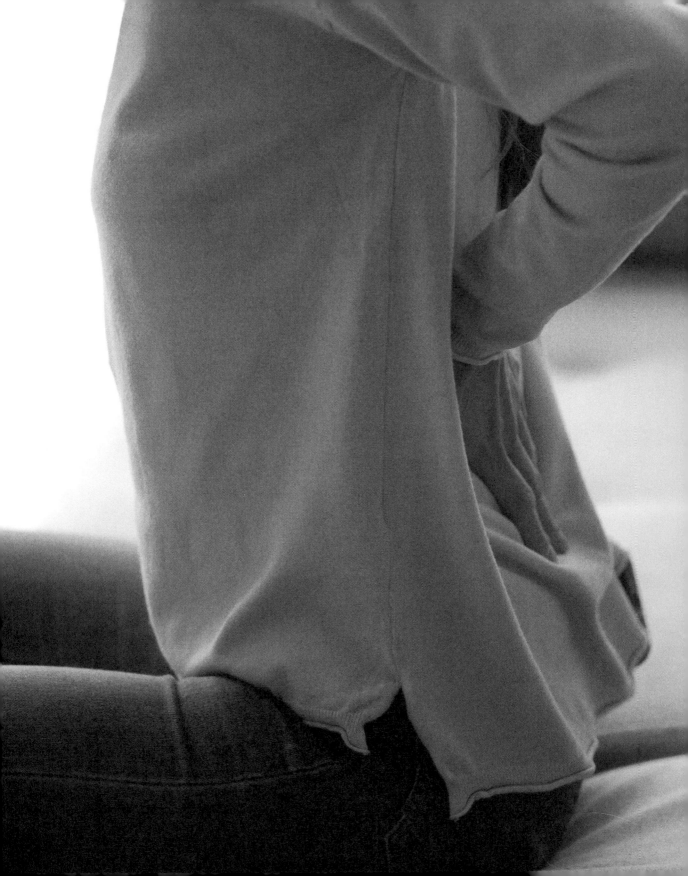

CHAPTER 3

Common back problems

If your back hurts, you're certainly not alone. Most adults experience at least one episode of back pain during their lifetimes, and many people deal with back pain on a frequent basis. Back-related problems are one of the most common reasons people see their doctors.

Your back serves three main functions — to support the weight of your body, protect your spinal cord and spinal nerves, and facilitate movement, such as bending and twisting. A carefully arranged framework of bones (vertebrae), disks, joints, ligaments, tendons and muscles work in unison to make this happen.

When you consider all the work that your back does and the many components that keep it functioning, it's not surprising problems can arise. As you get older, changes in your spine often make your back more vulnerable to damage or injury. With age, parts of your spine can degenerate. Bones can wear away, become more brittle and fracture more easily. Rubbery disks can dry out and thin, leaving less cushioning between bones. Muscles, ligaments and tendons can stretch, loosen and weaken.

And because the structures that form your back work so closely together, a problem in one area can set off a chain reaction. For example, when a disk ruptures, its gel-like center may push into your spinal canal, narrowing the canal. With less space in the canal, your spinal nerves may become compressed. In addition to pain, you may experience tingling, numbness and weakness.

It's also not uncommon for back pain to occur without an identifiable cause. Of people who seek help for back problems, in many cases a doctor isn't able to make a specific diagnosis. This is known as nonspecific low back pain.

The good news is, most back pain — even when the cause is unknown — lasts only a short time, often several days to a few weeks. And in the majority of cases, the pain can be relieved with conservative treatments. Only rarely is surgery necessary to treat a back condition.

The conditions discussed in this chapter focus mainly on the lower section of your back, called the lumbar spine. The lumbar spine allows for a much greater degree of movement than the relatively stable upper and middle sections of your back, making your lower back more susceptible to injury. Conditions affecting the cervical spine — the neck — are detailed in the next chapter.

MUSCLE-RELATED CONDITIONS

Your back is made up of various ligaments, tendons and muscles that help you lift, pull, push, walk and sit. Your back muscles are among the muscles that supply nerves to your body, making them a potential source of back pain.

Ligaments and tendons are bands of fibrous tissue with separate functions. Ligaments hold vertebrae and disks together and prevent excessive joint movement, while tendons connect muscles to bone. These fibrous bands become thicker and less flexible as you age, making them more susceptible to injury.

Sprains and strains

Up to 90% of low back pain can be traced back to a strain or sprain in a muscle, ligament or tendon that supports the spine. The low back is a common site of injury because of its dual functions — to support the weight of the upper body while at the same time allowing for movement, such as twisting and bending. Though usually not serious, pain from these types of injuries can be debilitating.

A muscle strain occurs when muscle or tendon fibers are overstretched or torn due to overuse. A sprain, meanwhile, is the result of an injury that tears ligaments from their attachments. Sprains and strains may occur suddenly — for example, picking up an object that's too heavy, falling or moving awkwardly. Having an uncoordinated golf swing is one example of an awkward movement. Sprains and strains may also occur from seemingly harmless events, such as setting down a cup of coffee on a table or opening a door, particularly if you have a history of back problems.

In addition, sprains and strains can result from repetitive actions you might experience while working on an assembly line or loading or unloading boxes. Obesity, poor posture and a lack of regular exercise increase your risk of experiencing a sprain or strain.

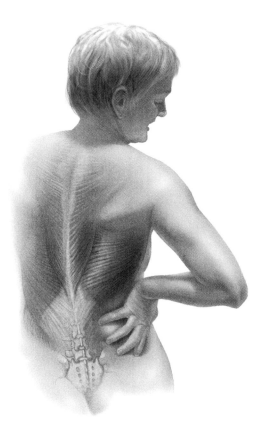

Sprains and strains. Lower back strains and sprains are the most common causes of back pain. Muscle strain results when muscle fibers are stretched or torn. Sprains occur when ligaments are torn from their attachments.

With both a sprain or strain, soft tissues become inflamed, causing pain and swelling. In general, you may be experiencing a sprain or strain in your lower back if you have:

- Short-term discomfort or soreness (two weeks or less)
- Pain that radiates into the buttocks but doesn't affect the legs

- Stiffness that limits your normal range of motion
- Problems sitting or standing upright
- A popping or tearing feeling in your back
- Muscle spasms that occur with or without activity

When dealing with a back strain or sprain, the last thing you probably feel like doing is moving. But staying active and out of bed is the best way to recover from these types of injuries. Long periods of bed rest can worsen your symptoms and cause you to lose muscle strength. Strong muscles are important to help support your spine.

Pain stemming from a sprain or strain can often be treated with over-the-counter non-steroidal anti-inflammatory pain relievers, such as ibuprofen (Advil, Motrin IB, others) and naproxen sodium (Aleve). Applying heat and ice to the painful area to reduce inflammation and loosen tight muscles, along with stretching exercises and massage, also may improve your symptoms.

Most sprains and strains heal within a month. If the pain lingers, your doctor may recommend physical therapy or specific interventional therapies. In case of a severe injury, surgery may be necessary to fix complete tears or separations.

Muscle spasms

A muscle spasm is a sudden, involuntary tightening of a muscle, usually in response to injury or overuse. You may experience the feeling of sudden, painful tightening. This feeling may last seconds or minutes or for days, and the pain can be debilitating.

Bending and twisting of your lower back, such as lifting a heavy object and turning to place it on a shelf, can strain your back muscles and the ligaments attached to them. If your muscle conditioning is poor, this can trigger painful muscle spasms.

Muscle spasms usually aren't serious and they often improve quickly with simple measures, such as rest, massage, stretching and daily exercise.

Sometimes, frequent spasms can indicate that something more serious is happening. For example, narrowing of the spinal canal (spinal stenosis) or a severe herniated disk can irritate or damage nerves within your back muscles, triggering a severe spasm.

Pain associated with a muscle spasm can often be relieved with ice and heat. Apply ice to the area up to four times a day for 20 minutes at a time to reduce inflammation. Do this the first couple of days. After you've iced the painful location, apply heat for 10 minutes at a time, as needed. Heat helps loosen and relax stiff muscles. A hot bath or shower can address more widespread pain.

Myofascial pain

Surrounding your back muscles is a layer of connective tissue known as fascia. This cov-

---

BY THE DEGREE

Sprains are sometimes described in terms of "degrees." A first-degree sprain causes only minor microscopic tearing of ligaments, resulting in a little tenderness and some pain. On the other end of the spectrum, a third-degree sprain is the complete tearing of the ligament. The pain is more severe and the joint that the injured ligament supports may become unstable.

Strains also are described by degree. A first-degree strain may produce minor pain and movement issues, while a third-degree strain involves the complete separation of a muscle from other muscles or tendons, or separation of one or more tendons from bone. There may also be bruising and loss of strength in the muscles.

ering attaches to major muscles in the abdomen, forming a multilayer "brace" for your abdominal and back muscles. Having this added support is particularly helpful when lifting objects.

When a back muscle is continually tightened (contracted) — often from overuse or repetitive motions — the fascia covering the muscle can become damaged or feel tight. However, just like a sprain or strain, even ordinary movements can trigger fascial tightening or damage. If you were to press on the affected area, you might feel a tight knot that's tender. Touching the sensitive area might also trigger a pattern of alternating spasms and pain.

This is known as myofascial pain. The pain develops in one or more spots along a muscle. These concentrated areas are called trigger points. Sometimes, the pain can travel to other, seemingly unrelated parts of the body. A crucial difference between myofascial pain and a sprain or strain is that myofascial pain often worsens with time.

Very focused areas of pain (trigger points) are the most common symptoms of myofascial pain. Less often you may experience:
• Muscle stiffness
• Headaches
• Fatigue

Myofascial pain can mimic symptoms of fibromyalgia, another condition also defined by pain and tenderness. Unlike myofascial pain, pain associated with fibromyalgia is generally more widespread and accompanied by other symptoms such as fatigue and sleep and mood issues. However, it may be possible to have both myofascial pain and fibromyalgia.

No one treatment is considered the gold standard for relieving myofascial pain. Treatment focuses on addressing trigger points. Options include physical therapy, pain medications, massage, stretching exercises and acupuncture. Needling is another treatment method in which a doctor inserts a thin needle in and around the trigger point to help break up muscle tension. Sometimes, a numbing agent or medication is injected during needling to help relieve pain.

DISK CONDITIONS

Located between each of the vertebrae in your back are small, rubbery cushions known as disks. Disks are flat, round and about one-half inch thick. Their main function is to act as shock absorbers, cushioning the impact to your back during activities such as walking, running or jumping. Disks also keep bone from rubbing on bone, and they help maintain the spine's height.

Disks can become damaged, often from wear and tear due to a physically demanding job or from degenerative changes that occur as we age. All people experience disk degeneration in varying degrees, often beginning with small tears in the outer edge of a disk. In some individuals, the degeneration becomes more extensive, causing problems.

Ruptured (herniated) disk

The disks in your spine contain a soft, gel-like core (nucleus). Surrounding this soft center is a protective outer layer of fiber (annulus) that keeps the core in place. When healthy, the gel-like core acts as a shock absorber, compressing when pressure or a load is placed upon your spine and relaxing when the load is removed.

With time, spinal disks lose a good portion of the water that forms the soft interior, and the protective outer layer stiffens. The result is that the outer layer of tissue bulges out fairly evenly all the way around its circumference, much like a hamburger that's too big for its bun. This is referred to as a bulging disk.

Eventually, tears may develop in the bulging outer layer, and the gel-like interior may protrude out of the disk. This is a herniated disk, which you may also hear described as a ruptured or slipped disk.

You're more at risk of experiencing a ruptured disk if you have a physically demanding job that involves bending, twisting or heavy lifting, or if you're overweight. Added weight places extra stress on your spine. Individuals who smoke also may be at increased risk because smoking reduces oxygen in blood, hastening disk breakdown.

Bulging disks are common and usually don't cause symptoms. Many people who have a ruptured disk don't know they have one. Sometimes, however, a ruptured disk

Normal   **Herniated disk**

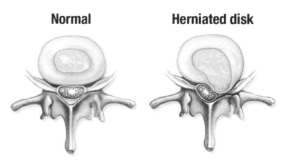

Herniation. When a spinal disk ruptures, its gel-like interior protrudes out from the center, creating a bulge (protrusion) in the disk's outer layer. The bulge may press on a nerve, causing pain (see the red on right image).

---

can irritate or press on a nearby nerve. Depending on where the rupture is located and the nerves involved, you may experience one or more of the following symptoms, usually affecting just one side of your body:

- **Pain.** If you have a ruptured disk in your lower back, you'll typically feel the most pain in your buttocks, thigh and calf. You might have pain in part of your foot, as well. The pain might shoot into your leg when you cough, sneeze or move into certain positions. The pain is often described as sharp or burning.
- **Numbness or tingling.** A ruptured disk may cause radiating numbness or tingling in parts of the body served by the affected nerves, including the buttocks and lower extremities.
- **Weakness.** Muscles served by the affected nerves may weaken, causing you to stumble or experience other difficulties walking or standing.

Pain from a ruptured disk typically improves over time as your body breaks down and absorbs the excess disk material, relieving pressure on adjacent nerves. Conservative treatment — mainly reducing activities that cause pain and taking over-the-counter pain medication — relieves symptoms in most people within a few days or weeks. Other options may include exercise, physical therapy and an injection of a steroid into the affected area, known as an epidural injection.

Few people with a ruptured disk need surgery. Your doctor might suggest surgery if conservative treatments fail to improve your symptoms, especially if you continue to have poorly controlled pain, numbness or weakness, difficulty standing or walking, or loss of bladder or bowel control. In most cases, a surgeon will remove just the protruding portion of the disk. Rarely, the entire disk is removed.

In some instances, a ruptured disk can cause severe spinal cord compression or cauda equina syndrome. These are medical emergencies and surgery may be needed to avoid permanent weakness or paralysis.

Disk collapse

At birth, spinal disks are composed mostly of water. With age, they gradually dehydrate. As you get older, your spinal disks may start to break down. As the disks thin, the bones in your spine begin to move closer together, causing your spine to lose height. This is one reason why we become a little shorter as we age.

Disk breakdown occurs to some degree in everyone; sort of like reading glasses, over time we all need them. Eventually, the tough outer wall of a disk may give out and the disk becomes flat. This is called a collapsed disk. Unlike a herniated disk, the inner core doesn't leak out.

Age is the biggest factor for disk collapse, although trauma is another potential cause. Not everyone will experience symptoms, particularly if the loss in disk height is mild. Sometimes, though, disk collapse can lead to bone rubbing on bone, spinal instability, and narrowing of the spinal canal and compression of spinal nerves. A collapsed disk may also place added stress on spinal joints, triggering deterioration.

Symptoms of disk collapse may include:
- A dull ache in the back
- Pressure across the lower back
- Pain that radiates to areas such as the buttocks, tailbone or thighs

Treatment typically consists of reducing activities that cause pain, pain medications, exercise, physical therapy and spinal injections. In severe cases, surgery may be necessary to replace the disk or stabilize the spine.

DEGENERATIVE DISEASE

Time, age, and normal wear and tear can damage the structures that make up your spine, leading to pain and discomfort. Degenerative disease is the term for back problems resulting from such changes. Degenerative disease can affect all parts of your spine, including vertebrae, disks, joints and ligaments.

Not everyone experiences these age-related changes, but for those who do, the pain can be severe.

Arthritis

There are many forms of arthritis. The most common is osteoarthritis. It occurs when cartilage breaks down or wears away at the end of a bone where the bone forms a joint. In the spine, osteoarthritis often affects the facet joints, where vertebrae join together. Often, the entire joint is affected, causing changes in the bone and deterioration of the connective tissues that hold the joint together and that attach muscle to bone. Osteoarthritis can also cause inflammation of the joint lining.

Multiple changes in the structure of your back that occur over time can lead to arthritis. Soft disks that provide cushioning between your bones can dry out and shrink, and the joints (facets) between the bones that allow the spine to move and twist can lose protective cartilage. The result is a narrowing of the space between the vertebrae, causing bone-on-bone friction and irritation.

Your body's response to degenerative arthritis often is to create bony outgrowths

(bone spurs) in an attempt to strengthen your spine. In some cases, bone spurs can narrow the spinal canal and pinch a nerve root.

A number of factors increase your risk of developing osteoarthritis, including older age, obesity, prior joint injury, repeated stress and a family history of arthritis. Females also are more likely to develop osteoarthritis, though it isn't clear why.

Pain is the most common symptom of back arthritis. When the pain first develops, you may notice that your discomfort is worse when you're active and that it improves with rest. Eventually, the pain may become constant. You may also experience:
- Limited range of motion
- Stiffness
- Swelling and tenderness near the affected vertebrae
- A grinding sensation when you bend or move your spine

Maintaining a healthy weight to reduce stress on your back can help reduce symptoms of arthritis. Other treatments include exercise — especially water-based activities that reduce strain on weight-bearing joints — physical therapy and over-the-counter pain medications. Some individuals may benefit from injections of steroid medications into painful areas. For severe pain that doesn't respond to conservative measures, prescription medications or procedures that short-circuit irritated nerves, such as radiofrequency ablation, may be prescribed. Rarely is surgery necessary.

OTHER TYPES OF ARTHRITIS

Osteoarthritis isn't the only type of arthritis that can cause back pain. Spondyloarthropathies is the name for a group of arthritic conditions that can lead to back problems. These forms of arthritis are different from other types in that they're specific to the locations where ligaments and tendons attach to bone:

- **Ankylosing spondylitis.** This form of chronic inflammatory arthritis affects the joint that connects the bone at the bottom of the spine to the pelvis (sacroiliac joint).
- **Psoriatic arthritis.** About 20% of people who have psoriatic arthritis — a type of arthritis that affects the joints and skin — also have spinal arthritis. For some, bone overgrowth can cause multiple vertebrae to grow or fuse together, which can result in stiffness.
- **Reactive arthritis.** Genital, urinary or gastrointestinal infections can sometimes trigger joint inflammation, including joints in the spine.
- **Enteropathic arthritis.** A small percentage of people with inflammatory bowel disease (ulcerative colitis and Crohn's disease) may experience enteropathic arthritis, which typically affects the sacroiliac joint.

In addition to pain, these forms of inflammatory arthritis often produce swelling or stiffness in other areas of the body — not just your back or neck.

Facet joint disease

Your spine owes much of its flexibility to what are known as facet joints. These small, stabilizing joints are located where one vertebra connects to the next. The joints are found in pairs along the back of your spine, on each level of vertebrae. The facet joints help keep your spine aligned as it moves, and they allow the spine to flex, extend and rotate.

As is the case with any joint in your body, age and natural wear and tear can affect the joints, causing pain. Facet joint disease results from a breakdown of cartilage that covers and protects the ends of the joints. As the cartilage deteriorates, bone can rub on bone. This may lead to a pointed outgrowth of bone known as a bone spur or to enlargement of the joint. Both of these conditions can irritate and compress adjacent nerves.

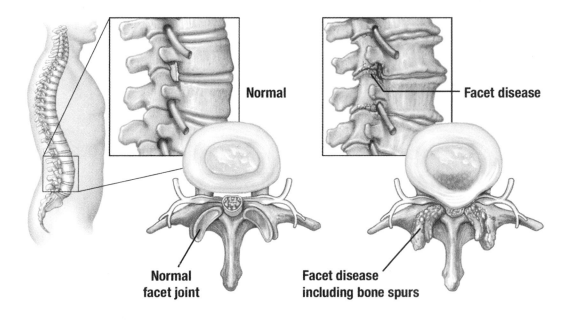

Normal

Facet disease

Normal facet joint

Facet disease including bone spurs

Facet disease. Facet disease, also called facet syndrome, is a painful degeneration of the facet joints in the spine. The facet joints connect vertebrae together.

It's not uncommon to see facet joint disease alongside other conditions, such as disk collapse and narrowing of the spinal canal (spinal stenosis).

Pain and stiffness are the hallmarks of facet joint disease. These symptoms are usually felt near the affected joint. The pain is often worse after a period of inactivity or sleep. In some individuals, the pain may radiate to other parts of the body, such as a buttock, hip or thigh.

Age, a history of spinal trauma, degenerative disk disease, poor posture and a family history of degenerative arthritis all increase your risk of developing facet joint disease.

Treatment for facet joint disease focuses on relieving pain and stiffness and helping you to stay as active as possible.

Over-the-counter anti-inflammatory medications, such as ibuprofen (Advil, Motrin IB, others) or naproxen sodium (Aleve), and applying heat or ice to the painful area may relieve your discomfort. Physical therapy is often recommended to help treat facet joint disease, focusing on stretching and strengthening your abdominal and lower back muscles. When conservative treatments aren't helpful, an injection of a steroid into your spine or other nonsurgical approaches may be recommended, including procedures to destroy nerve fibers carrying pain signals.

SYNOVIAL CYST

Sometimes, degeneration of a facet joint can lead to the development of a fluid-filled growth that forms in the joint, called a synovial cyst. When a cyst forms, it may compress nerve roots exiting from the joint, causing pain and other symptoms.

Synovial cysts are thought to develop when there's an unusually large range of motion in the spine. The exaggerated motion may place increased stress on the facet joints, resulting in an accumulation of excess fluid in the joint.

If a synovial cyst isn't causing any problems, your doctor may recommend observation to see if the cyst shrinks or enlarges. It you're experiencing symptoms, treatment may include pain-relief medications, physical therapy or an injection at the location of the cyst. If symptoms persist, surgery may be necessary to remove the cyst.

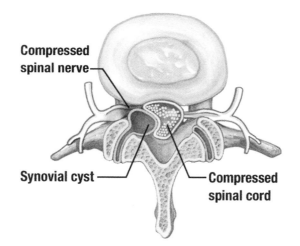

Synovial cyst. A synovial cyst is a fluid-filed sac that develops along the spine. Most synovial cysts don't cause symptoms, but sometimes a cyst may press on nerve roots or the spinal cord, causing pain and other symptoms.

Grades of spondylolisthesis

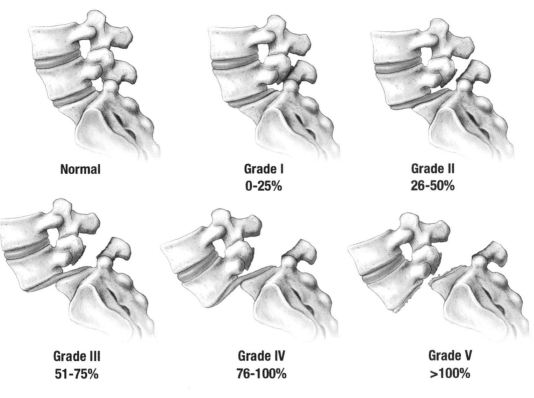

Normal

Grade I
0-25%

Grade II
26-50%

Grade III
51-75%

Grade IV
76-100%

Grade V
>100%

Spondylolisthesis. Spondylolisthesis can be described according to its degree of severity, with grade I being least advanced and grade V being the most advanced. The grade is determined by measuring how much of a vertebral body has slipped forward over the body beneath it.

Spondylosis and spondylolisthesis

Spondylosis is a catch-all medical term used to describe general age-related wear and tear on all structures of the spine. It's an alternative to the label "nonspecific low back pain" and a common diagnosis in older adults who typically have multiple degenerative diseases that could trigger pain. Spondylosis is commonly seen alongside conditions such as spinal stenosis, arthritis, bone spurs and spondylolisthesis.

The term *spondylolisthesis* refers to instability in the spine, typically caused by one vertebra shifting onto an adjacent vertebra and pinching adjoining nerves. Spondylolisthesis may be triggered by a spinal fracture or spinal instability stemming from joint or disk disease.

Among people with spondylolisthesis, the severity of symptoms is often linked to the degree to which one or more vertebrae have shifted. These degrees are referred to medically as grades. Generally, individuals with the most slippage have the worst pain.

Signs and symptoms associated with spondylosis and spondylolisthesis are often worse with activity and improve with rest. They include:

- Discomfort similar to a muscle strain
- Back stiffness
- Tenderness in the affected area
- Sudden tightening of muscles (spasms)
- Reduced range of motion
- Lower back pain that radiates to the buttocks and back of the thighs
- Numbness or weakness in the legs
- Problems walking or standing for long periods

Treatment typically focuses on relieving the pain. This may include use of over-the-counter pain relievers such as ibuprofen (Advil, Motrin IB, others) and naproxen sodium (Aleve), as well as exercise and physical therapy. In cases where these treatments are ineffective and symptoms persist, surgery may be necessary to stabilize the spine.

NERVE-RELATED CONDITIONS

Your spine serves as the main passageway for your spinal cord. The spinal cord is a rope-like column of nerves that links your brain to the nerves in your arms, legs and trunk. It's surrounded by the small bones (vertebrae) that compose your spinal column.

The spinal cord contains a total of 31 pairs of nerves. Each of these pairs branches off of the spinal cord between each vertebra, forming nerve roots. If your spinal cord or one of these roots becomes compressed or damaged, pain can occur.

Pinched or damaged nerve

Due to the intricate composition of your spine, when one spinal condition develops a cascade of other problems can follow, often affecting a nerve. For example, a ruptured (herniated) disk can press on a nerve root near where the nerve exits the spine and branches to the legs. The disk pinches the nerve, resulting in pain, and often numbness and tingling. Bone spurs, narrowing of the spinal canal and tumors can press on spinal nerves and cause pain.

The medical term for radiating pain due to a pinched or damaged nerve is radiculitis. Radiating nerve pain accompanied by neurologic symptoms such as numbness or weakness is called radiculopathy.

Other conditions that can cause nerve damage include trauma, a bone infection and diabetes. A ruptured disk also may release a chemical that's irritating to the nerve root, triggering pain and associated symptoms.

A pinched or damaged nerve can produce a variety of signs and symptoms, depending on the part of the spine that is affected:

- Sharp pain, typically on one side of the body, that radiates to a buttock and leg
- Numbness or tingling in a buttock and leg

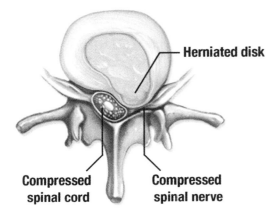

Herniated disk

Compressed spinal cord

Compressed spinal nerve

Pinched (compressed) nerve. A pinched nerve occurs when too much pressure is applied to a nerve. A herniated disk may put pressure on a nerve root, compressing the nerve and causing pain and other symptoms.

- Pain that worsens with certain actions, such as coughing or sneezing, or with prolonged sitting or walking
- Weakness or loss of reflexes in a hip, knee, foot or ankle
- Trouble walking, including stumbling
- Bladder and bowel control problems

Unlike other forms of back pain, conservative treatments such as over-the-counter pain medications or cold and heat therapy often aren't helpful for radiculopathy. Prescription medications that target the nervous system, such as anticonvulsants and tricyclic antidepressants seem to work best to improve symptoms.

Steroid injections, when used in conjunction with an exercise or a rehabilitation program,

also may improve symptoms. Surgery is typically reserved for people still experiencing pain after other treatments have failed, and those whose neurologic symptoms are severe or worsening.

Spinal stenosis

The spinal canal is the circular, open space inside the vertebral column that houses and protects the spinal cord. In most people, the spinal cord passes through the canal unhindered. However, age and wear and tear can produce multiple changes that may cause the spinal canal to narrow. Narrowing of the spinal canal is called spinal stenosis.

Some people are born with a small spinal canal, but most cases of spinal stenosis occur when something happens to narrow the open space. Bone spurs are a common cause of spinal stenosis. Bone spurs are bone overgrowths that can result from wear and tear. These growths can take up valuable space within the spinal canal and place pressure on the nerves that travel through the spine. Compression of the nerves in the lower spine is called neurogenic claudication.

Spinal stenosis and neurogenic claudication can also result from other causes. Sometimes a severely herniated disk that presses on the spinal cord is the culprit. Tumors, thickened ligaments and spinal injuries also can lead to narrowing of the spinal canal.

Not everyone who has spinal stenosis experiences symptoms. Signs and symptoms

SCIATICA

Sciatica is a form of radiculopathy caused by compression of the sciatic nerve. The sciatic nerve is a large nerve that branches from your lower back through your hips and buttocks and down the back of each leg.

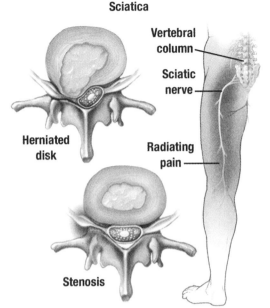

Sciatica

Vertebral column

Sciatic nerve

Herniated disk

Radiating pain

Stenosis

Compression of the sciatic nerve can lead to varying degrees of pain, from a mild ache to shock-like pain or a burning sensation. Sciatica may also cause numbness and tingling. These symptoms typically occur only on one side of the body, and they extend down the lower back and thigh to the ankle or foot. In severe cases, sciatica may cause muscle weakness in a leg or foot. Loss of bowel and bladder control also may occur.

Age-related changes in the spine, including a herniated disk, a bone spur or narrowing of the spinal canal (spinal stenosis), are the most common causes of sciatica. However, anything that puts additional stress on your back can increase your risk, including obesity, a physically demanding job and prolonged sitting. Diabetes increases your risk of nerve damage and, in turn, sciatica.

Although the pain associated with sciatica can be severe, most cases resolve within weeks with conservative treatments, including application of cold and heat, stretching, and over-the-counter pain relievers. In some cases, a doctor may recommend physical therapy, a steroid injection or prescription medications. People with severe sciatica associated with significant leg weakness or bowel or bladder changes might be candidates for surgery to remove the structure causing the compression, such as a herniated disk or bone spur.

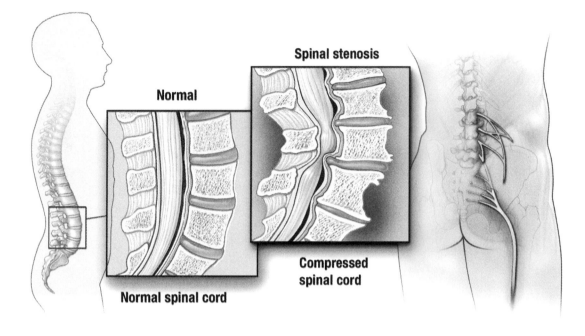

Spinal stenosis. Spinal stenosis is a narrowing of the spaces within your spine, which can put pressure on the nerves that travel through the spine, including the spinal cord.

---

generally occur when spinal nerves become compressed. They may include:

- Numbness or tingling in a foot or leg
- Weakness in a foot or leg
- Pain worsened by walking or standing for long periods and relieved by bending forward or sitting
- Back pain

Treatment for spinal stenosis depends on the location of the narrowing (stenosis) and the severity of your symptoms. Individuals with mild to moderate symptoms may benefit from physical therapy, medications or steroid injections. An exercise program that focuses on strengthening back and abdominal muscles also may be beneficial. Surgery may be considered if other treatments haven't helped or your symptoms are severe.

Cauda equina syndrome

At the end of your spinal cord is a bundle of 18 nerves that looks like a horse's tail. Called the cauda equina, the Latin words for horse's tail, these nerves are tasked with sending and receiving nerve signals to and from the pelvic organs and lower limbs.

A variety of conditions, such as a herniated disk, trauma, a tumor or an infection, can compress or damage cauda equina nerves. If two or more of the nerves are compressed, in addition to back pain you may experience issues affecting sensation and movement, as well as bladder, bowel and sexual health issues. This cluster of symptoms is known as cauda equina syndrome.

Although rare, cauda equina syndrome is a medical emergency requiring surgery shortly after the onset of symptoms to remove the source of the compression and lessen the risk of paralysis and permanent damage.

Signs and symptoms of cauda equina syndrome can vary in severity and may develop gradually. Signs and symptoms may include the following:

- Severe low back pain
- Weakness, loss of sensation, or pain in one or both legs
- Numbness between the legs, buttocks, inner thighs, back of the legs and feet
- Urinary incontinence or retention
- Bowel incontinence
- Sexual dysfunction
- Loss of reflexes in the legs

Unfortunately, even if you're treated immediately, recovery of specific functions can take months or even years, and there's no guarantee that these functions will ever fully return to normal.

JOINT INFLAMMATION

The joints that connect your lower spine to your pelvis are known as the sacroiliac joints. They are some of the largest joints in your body. The sacroiliac joints help distribute body weight from your lower spine to your pelvis. When these joints are damaged, they can become inflamed, triggering pain — a condition called sacroiliitis.

Sacroiliitis

Common causes for sacroiliac joint damage include trauma from an accident or fall, various types of arthritis — including wear-and-tear arthritis (osteoarthritis) and inflammatory arthritis (ankylosing spondylitis) — pregnancy, and infection.

The symptoms of sacroiliitis can mimic other sources of back pain, making its diagnosis tricky. In fact, the condition is often overlooked as a potential cause of back pain. Sacroiliitis triggers pain in the lower back or buttocks, sometimes extending down one or both legs. Pain may also occur in the groin and feet and trigger muscle spasms. The pain may fall on either end of the spectrum — dull and achy or sharp and stabbing. It may worsen when you:

- Stand for long periods
- Climb stairs
- Bear more weight on one leg than the other
- Run
- Take long strides

Over-the-counter pain medications can help relieve the pain, but some people need stronger prescription medications. Physical therapy, steroids injections and procedures

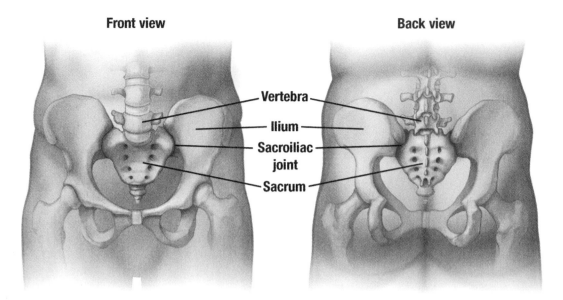

Front view   **Back view**

Vertebra

Ilium

Sacroiliac
joint

Sacrum

Sacroiliitis. Sacroiliitis is an inflammation of one or both of your sacroiliac joints — situated where your lower spine and pelvis connect. Sacroiliitis can cause pain in your buttocks or lower back, and can extend down one or both legs.

that destroy the pain-causing nerves (radiofrequency denervation) also may bring relief. Surgery is rarely necessary to treat sacroiliitis. Most people with the condition get relief from their symptoms within a few weeks, although recurrence is common.

SPINAL DEFORMITIES

If you were to look at a healthy spine from the side, you'd notice that the spinal vertebrae form a gentle S-curve. This shape allows for even distribution of your weight and for flexibility of movement. When you look at your spine from the back, its bones form a relatively straight line. When your spine loses this natural alignment back pain can occur. Scoliosis is one example.

Scoliosis

Scoliosis is a sideways curvature of your spine and a common spinal deformity. When viewed from behind, the spine appears to be curved, or shifted, to one side instead of straight. Most cases of scoliosis are mild, but some can be severe.

Scoliosis-related back pain usually doesn't appear until middle age. And people with scoliosis who experience pain often have another underlying condition, such as spon-

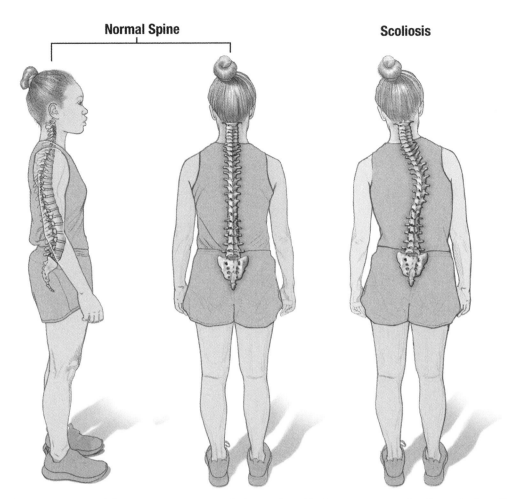

Normal Spine   **Scoliosis**

Scoliosis. Scoliosis is a sideways curvature of the spine that occurs most often during the growth spurt just before puberty.

dylolisthesis, a herniated disk or a spinal tumor contributing to the problem.

Most often, the cause of scoliosis isn't known, although it may be hereditary because it tends to run in families. Less commonly, conditions such as cerebral palsy, muscular dystrophy, birth defects, or spinal injuries or infections may cause scoliosis.

Most individuals with the disease are born with an abnormal curvature of the spine and are diagnosed during childhood or adolescence. Adults with scoliosis typically fall into three categories: They were unsuccessfully treated for scoliosis as children; they never received treatment as children; or they have a condition called degenerative scoliosis.

Degenerative scoliosis usually occurs in the lower back in people age 65 and older. It's sometimes accompanied by narrowing of the spinal canal (spinal stenosis). Back pain from degenerative scoliosis may develop very gradually and you may notice it only when you're active.

Changes to the spine that occur in degenerative scoliosis may be very minor and not apparent by just looking at the spine. But there are other clues:

- Your shoulders, rib cage, hips or waist are uneven
- Your head isn't centered directly above your pelvis
- Your body leans to one side
- The shape or size of your chest is abnormal, which can affect breathing

Adults with scoliosis may experience mild to significant progression of their symptoms. Surgery typically is only recommended for a severe curvature of the spine, or if the condition is causing neurologic problems, such as difficulty walking or incontinence.

TRAUMA AND FRACTURES

Most spinal fractures occur in one of three places: the middle of the spine (thoracic spine), the lower back (lumbar spine) or the location where these two connect, an area called the thoracolumbar junction.

Some fractures are considered stable, meaning they usually don't require surgery. An example is a fracture caused by thinning bones (osteoporosis). Stable fractures may develop gradually and not cause any symptoms until the bone breaks. Unstable fractures are those that require surgery to realign the bone. Unstable fractures are more common in cases of trauma such as an accident or fall.

Accidents and injuries

Your spine is actually quite resilient and can handle a significant amount of stress. However, an event such as a car accident or a fall off of a ladder can fracture a vertebra. Spinal fractures can range from mild to life-threatening.

Spinal fractures are classified by the pattern of the fracture and whether the spinal cord is involved:

- **Axial burst fracture.** It causes the vertebrae to collapse. This type of fracture is most common if you land on your feet after falling from considerable height.
- **Chance (flexion/distraction) fracture.** It occurs when the vertebrae are pulled apart — usually in a car accident, especially if your body is sent flying forward while your seat belt braces your pelvis.
- **Fracture-dislocation.** Trauma may cause one vertebra to separate from an adjacent vertebra. When this type of injury happens, the spinal cord may become compressed.

Fractures can cause moderate to severe back pain that worsens with activity. You may also experience numbness, tingling and weakness in your legs, and bowel or bladder problems with spinal cord compression.

Stable fractures often require wearing a back brace and avoiding certain activities while the bone heals. An unstable fracture may require surgery, especially if the damage is severe.

Osteoporosis

The bone-thinning disease osteoporosis can weaken bones in your spine, making them susceptible to fracture. If you have osteoporosis, even low-impact activities such as reaching for a box on a shelf or twisting to put on a seatbelt can result in a fracture. You may not know a fracture is developing in a vertebra until the bone actually breaks.

Osteoporosis is a common source of compression fractures, which cause the front of a vertebra to break and collapse, while leaving the back intact (see the illustration on page 56). Generally, the bone doesn't move, meaning it's usually a stable fracture and the compression doesn't cause neurologic problems such as tingling or numbness in the legs.

However, compression fractures can cause significant pain, particularly if you have three or more fractures. The pain may come on suddenly and radiate to the front of your body. It usually improves over the course of several weeks. However, once you've had a vertebral fracture your risk for future fractures is increased.

Stable fractures can often be treated conservatively. You may need to wear a brace for a few months and limit your activities. Other treatment for osteoporotic fractures includes medications to help promote bone growth and decrease pain. Engaging in weight-bearing exercises that help build bone also is beneficial, as is a nutritious and healthy diet.

INFECTIONS AND TUMORS

The vast majority of back pain can be attributed to conditions such as sprains and strains or to degenerative disease. Occasionally, back pain is associated with a less common cause. Infections can affect all structures of the spine. Tumors also can develop on the spine, causing pain.

Infections

Spinal infections, including infection in a vertebra or disk (diskitis), are relatively rare. A spinal infection needs to be treated quickly to reduce serious complications, including paralysis and death.

In about half of cases, a urinary tract infection is the source of a spinal infection. An infection may spread by way of arteries in the spine, extending from soft tissue to bones and disks. The infection can move quickly, advancing from where a vertebra

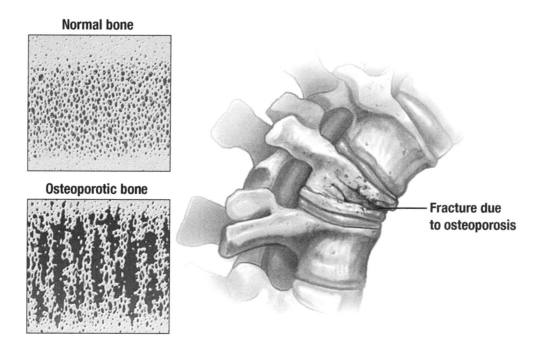

Normal bone

Osteoporotic bone

Fracture due to osteoporosis

Osteoporosis. Bone is living tissue that's constantly being broken down and replaced. Osteoporosis occurs when the creation of new bone doesn't keep up with the loss of old bone, causing bone to fracture.

and disk meet (end plates) into the disk and then on to neighboring vertebrae.

Symptoms of a spinal infection may include:
- Low back pain
- Radiating pain
- Pain that worsens and progresses with time

Antibiotics to control the infection are critical to treatment. Surgery usually isn't necessary unless the spine becomes unstable or you've developed specific neurologic problems. Damage to soft tissue may require surgery to remove dead tissue, known as surgical debridement.

Tumors

Though not a common source of back pain, tumors that grow on the spine can compress spinal nerves, causing pain and neurological problems. The tumor may be noncancerous or cancerous. However, spinal tumors of any variety can cause permanent disability and may be life-threatening.

There are several places where spinal tumors may develop. A tumor that forms within the spinal cord is called an intramedullary tumor. A tumor that develops on the covering of the spinal cord or the nerve roots that branch out from the cord is known as an extramedullary tumor. A tumor that affects the bones of the spine (vertebrae) is called a vertebral tumor.

It's not clear why most spinal tumors develop. Experts suspect that defective genes play a role, but whether such genetic defects are inherited or develop over time is often unknown. In some cases, a spinal cord tumor is linked to known inherited syndromes, such as neurofibromatosis 2 and von Hippel-Lindau disease.

It's not uncommon for cancer that develops in other parts of the body to spread (metastasize) to the vertebrae, the supporting network around the spinal cord or, in rare cases, the spinal cord itself. Two-thirds of people who are diagnosed with cancer will have a tumor that metastasizes. Among individuals with lung, breast, prostate or kidney cancer, the spine is a common place for these metastases to form.

Signs and symptoms of a spinal cord tumor may include:
- Pain at the site of the tumor
- Back pain that radiates to other parts of your body and is worse at night
- Reduced sensitivity to pain, heat and cold
- Difficulty walking, due to loss of sensation in your legs
- Muscle weakness
- Loss of bowel or bladder function

Back pain is a common early symptom of a spinal tumor. Any new onset of back pain that doesn't improve or that isn't relieved with rest should be evaluated by your doctor, especially if you have a history of cancer. Treatment for a spinal tumor may include surgery, radiation therapy, chemotherapy and other medications.

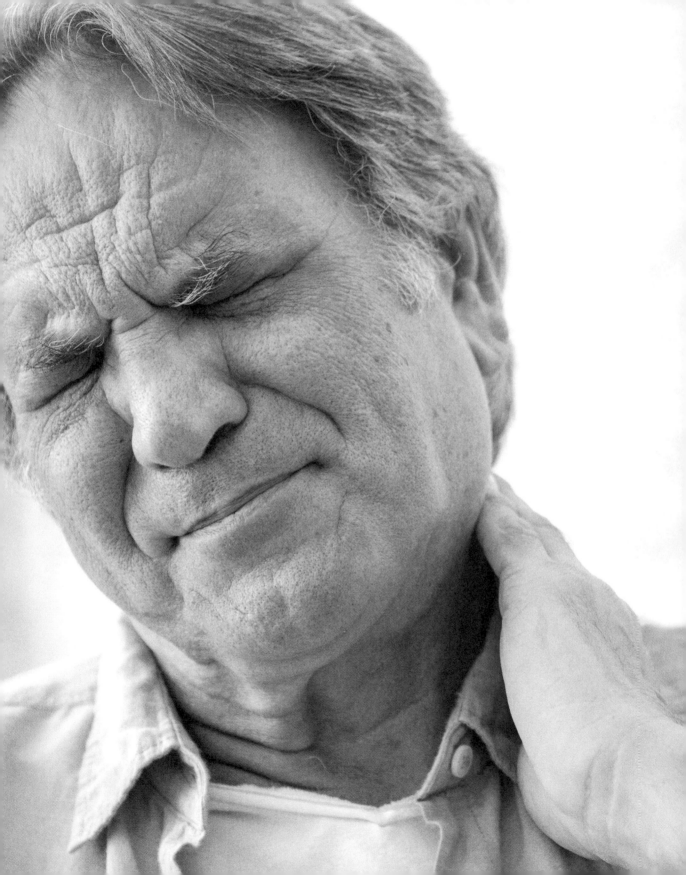

CHAPTER 4

Common neck problems

Your neck, like your back, provides the basic framework for your body to function. It supports the weight of your head and keeps it stable while remaining flexible enough to allow movement in multiple directions. The neck's cervical spine also helps protect the delicate spinal nerves that facilitate communication between your brain and the rest of your body. Unlike other areas of your spine, the cervical spine lacks significant protection, making it particularly vulnerable to injury and pain.

Neck pain is a common complaint. Many people have experienced neck pain at some point in their lives. It may be a dull soreness felt first thing in the morning after sleeping in an awkward position, or a more uncomfortable "zinging" pain that stops you in your tracks. In some cases, neck issues may trigger pain in other parts of the body, such as the shoulders, arms or hands. This is known as referred pain.

Often times, neck pain is temporary and gradually disappears with conservative treatment. Occasionally, the pain becomes chronic and requires more-intensive measures to relieve it.

Pain in your neck may arise for a number of reasons. Soft tissue injuries, such as sprains, strains and damaged nerves, are some of the most common causes of neck pain. Other types of pain may stem from disk damage, such as a ruptured (herniated) disk, or from degenerative conditions, such as arthritis. These problems are often interrelated, with one potentially triggering another. For example, a condition that causes narrowing of the spinal canal may produce nerve damage. Sometimes, the cause of the pain isn't known.

MUSCLE-RELATED CONDITIONS

The cervical spine is made up of an interconnected network of muscles and other soft tissues — ligaments and tendons — that hold together the vertebrae in your neck and keep the bones aligned. These soft tissues lend support to your neck while also giving it the ability to move up, down, side to side, forward and backward. When muscles, tendons and ligaments sustain injury, the resulting pain can range from mild to severe and last a short period (acute pain) or months or years (chronic pain).

Sprains and strains

Though the terms are often used interchangeably, sprains and strains affect different soft tissue. A cervical sprain results when ligaments in the neck are overstretched or torn. A strain is an injury to neck muscles and tendons, typically due to excessive stress placed on the neck. About 85% of neck pain can be traced back to sprains and strains. Pain that results from a sprain or strain can affect numerous areas, including the back of the head and shoulders.

Neck strain can occur for a variety of reasons. Common causes include poor posture, stress-related muscle tension and poor sleep habits. Sprains are often caused by sudden trauma to the neck, such as an auto accident or fall, or they may be due to a sports injury. Sometimes, however, a seemingly harmless action, such as turning your head when someone calls your name or stretching your

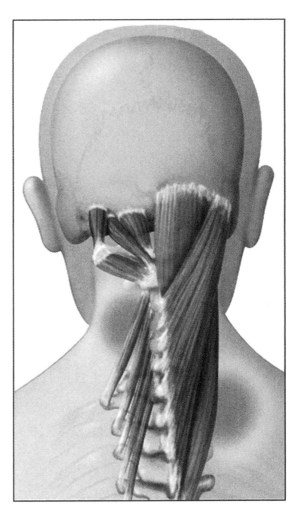

Sprains and strains. Neck sprains and strains are common. They result when ligaments, tendons and muscles are stretched too far or torn or when stress-related tension develops in a muscle.

neck to see around something in front of you, can produce a sprain or strain.

Neck pain also is linked to greater use of electronic devices such as cellphones, lap-

RARE NECK DISORDER

Cervical dystonia, also known as spasmodic torticollis, is a rare, painful condition in which your neck muscles contract uncontrollably, causing your head to twist or turn to one side. The condition also can cause your head to tilt forward or backward.

Cervical dystonia often occurs in middle-aged women, though it can affect people of any age and sex. In most cases, the cause of the condition isn't known, although a family history of the disorder increases your risk of developing it. Head, neck or shoulder injuries also are possible culprits.

There is no cure for cervical dystonia. Treatment focuses on relieving signs and symptoms.

top computers and tablets. Bending your neck to hold your cellphone to your ear or looking down at your phone, laptop or tablet for long periods can take your neck out of its normal position and stretch neck muscles and ligaments.

Discomfort from a neck sprain or strain can last several weeks. Common signs and symptoms include:
- Pain that worsens when you move your neck and shoulders
- Stiffness or limited range of motion
- Tightness in your upper back or shoulders
- Headaches

When you're dealing with a sprain or strain other problems can occur. You may have trouble sleeping. You may find it difficult to concentrate on tasks. You may not be able to take part in activities you enjoy. Sometimes — especially when the pain lingers — depression can result.

Neck sprains and strains often can be treated with conservative measures. They include use of nonsteroidal anti-inflammatory drugs (NSAIDs), such as ibuprofen (Advil, Motrin IB) and naproxen sodium (Aleve). Massage and applying heat or cold to the painful area several times a day for up to 20 minutes may help manage your symptoms. Cold helps reduce inflammation. Heat, including taking a warm shower or using a heating pad, helps relax tight muscles.

Muscle spasm

A muscle spasm is a sudden and uncontrolled tightening of a muscle that can occur when a muscle becomes fatigued or strained. Muscle spasms that occur in your neck are often reactions to everyday occurrences. Maybe you spent too long hunched over a computer screen or slept with your neck in an awkward position. Stress also can trigger muscle spasms.

Although generally harmless, neck spasms can be very painful and they also may trigger a headache. You may also find it difficult to move your neck. Treatment usually involves simple measures, such as rest and applying heat or cold to the painful area. Massage and neck exercises also may bring pain relief. For more-severe spasms, medication may be prescribed.

If you experience muscle spasms following an injury, such as a car accident that caused whiplash, you should see your doctor for a complete evaluation. Severe, frequent or persistent spasms may signal a more serious underlying condition, such as a muscle injury or a nerve or disk problem.

Myofascial pain syndrome

Following an injury, or if you overuse your muscles, tight fibers can form within the muscles. These sensitive areas are called trigger points. A trigger point in a muscle can cause strain and pain throughout the muscle. When this pain persists and worsens, doctors call it myofascial pain syndrome.

Cervical myofascial pain syndrome is a chronic pain disorder in which the layer of connective tissue surrounding the neck muscles (fascia) becomes damaged or feels tight. The condition typically occurs after a muscle is repeatedly tightened (contracted). This can happen when you perform repetitive motions involving your neck, such as a house painter who frequently looks up while painting.

Myofascial pain syndrome can also result from a neck injury or stress- or anxiety-related muscle tension that can lead to the development of a trigger point. Similar to a sprain or strain, even a seemingly harmless movement can trigger the disorder. Individuals with poor posture or deconditioned muscles are more at risk of developing myofascial pain syndrome.

Signs and symptoms may include:
- Tight, achy muscles in the neck
- Deep, aching pain that persists or worsens
- A tender knot in a muscle that's painful when you press on it
- Limited range of motion
- Pain that spreads from the neck to other parts of the body, such as the shoulders

Research suggests that for some individuals, myofascial pain syndrome may develop into fibromyalgia. Fibromyalgia is a disorder characterized by widespread musculoskeletal pain accompanied by fatigue, sleep, memory and mood issues. Fibromyalgia is

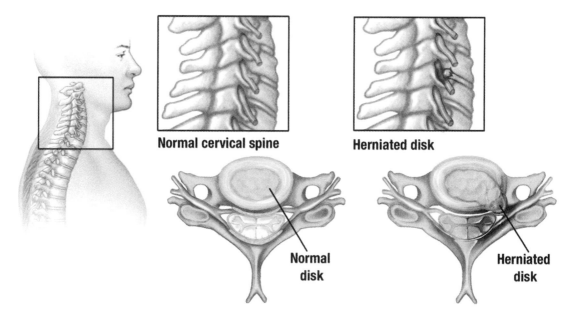

Normal cervical spine

Herniated disk

Normal disk

Herniated disk

Ruptured (herniated) disk. Spinal disks have a gel-like center encased in a tougher, rubbery exterior. A herniated disk occurs when some of the disk's gel-like material pushes out through a tear in the exterior wall. Pain can occur if the ruptured disk presses on adjacent nerves.

thought to be associated with increased sensitivity to pain signals within the body's central nervous system. Some doctors believe that myofascial pain syndrome may play a role in triggering this process.

Treatment for cervical myofascial pain syndrome includes physical therapy and injection of medication into sensitive trigger points. Pain medications and relaxation techniques also may be recommended.

DISK CONDITIONS

As you read in earlier chapters, the bones that make up your spine (vertebrae) are separated by rubbery cushions (disks) that are filled with a gel-like material. These disks allow the spine to move easily and serve as shock absorbers during activities. With age, these disks often become less flexible and more prone to tearing or rupture. Even with a minor strain or twist, the gel-like material inside a disk can push out (rupture) through its exterior. A ruptured disk can put pressure on the spinal cord and surrounding nerves, producing pain.

Wear and tear is the most common reason a disk will rupture. Trauma is another possible cause. You're also at increased risk of a ruptured disk if you're overweight or you work a physically demanding job. In addition, other medical conditions that affect your spine may place you at increased risk of disk damage. Oftentimes, it's difficult to pinpoint a specific reason or activity that triggered the problem.

Some people who have a ruptured cervical disk don't experience any symptoms, and it's only when an X-ray is taken for another condition that they learn of the problem. Others have mild to severe pain.

Depending on where the damaged disk is located, you may experience other symptoms that usually affect only one side of the body:

- **Shoulder and arm pain.** A ruptured disk in your neck can produce pain in your shoulder and arm. The pain might shoot down your arm to your hand when you cough, sneeze or move a certain way. The pain is often described as sharp or burning. In rare cases, when a ruptured cervical disk compresses the spinal cord, symptoms can develop in the legs, including difficulty walking.
- **Numbness or tingling.** A ruptured disk that presses on a nerve can cause numbness or a tingling sensation in the neck. These sensations can radiate to the shoulders, arms or hands.
- **Weakness.** Over time, arm and shoulder muscles served by the affected nerve can weaken. This may affect your ability to pick up or hold items.

Treatment for a ruptured cervical disk may include pain medication, injections of a steroid into the painful area (epidural injection) and physical therapy. Generally, surgery is necessary only if the rupture is severe.

DEGENERATIVE DISEASE

When in peak form, your neck is a master feat of anatomical engineering that allows you to bend and move your head in multiple directions. Over time, normal wear and tear on spinal structures, such as disks and joints, can damage the structures, leading to pain and discomfort.

Not everyone experiences these age-related changes, but for those who do, the pain can be severe.

Arthritis

Osteoarthritis is a common cause of neck pain. When you hear the word *arthritis* you may think of your knees, hips or back, and not your neck. However, many people develop arthritis in neck joints. Osteoarthritis of the neck is called cervical spondylosis, and it affects more than 85% of people age 60 and older.

In addition to age, other factors that increase your risk of neck arthritis include a previous neck injury, performing overhead or repetitive neck motions, and genetics — arthritis is more common in some families. If you smoke, you may be at an increased risk of neck arthritis. Research suggests that smoking can accelerate the breakdown of spinal disks.

A range of arthritis-related changes may lead to pain. The soft disks that provide cushioning between your bones (vertebrae) can dry out and shrink, and the joints (facets) between the bones that allow the cervical spine to move and twist can lose protective cartilage. The result is very little cushioning between the vertebrae and more bone-to-bone contact, causing friction and irritation.

Arthritis in the neck doesn't always cause pain. When signs and symptoms do occur, they may include:

- Mild to severe pain and stiffness, especially when you keep your head in the same position for extended periods of time
- Loss of flexibility in the neck
- Headaches
- A grinding or popping sensation when you turn your neck
- Numbness or weakness in your arms, hands and fingers
- Neck and shoulder spasms

Sometimes, neck arthritis results in a narrowing of the spinal canal that houses the spinal cord and nerve roots. If the spinal cord or nerve roots in the neck become pinched, you might experience tingling, numbness and weakness in your arms and hands, or even legs and feet. Other signs and symptoms can include lack of coordination and difficulty walking, or loss of bowel and bladder control. These signs and symptoms require immediate medical attention.

Rest and application of heat and cold to the painful area can often help reduce arthritis symptoms. Other treatments used to manage osteoarthritis of the neck include pain medication, joint injections and physical therapy.

Rheumatoid arthritis is a less common form of arthritis. Unlike osteoarthritis, it's an autoimmune disorder, meaning that the body's immune system turns on itself. Rheumatoid arthritis attacks the lining of the joints (synovium). Although rheumatoid arthritis is more common in other joints, it can affect the cervical spine.

Bone spurs

Over time, as the gel-like disks in your spine age and weaken, they may collapse, leaving less space and little cushioning between the bones of your neck. This puts increased pressure on the spine's facet joints, often resulting in a wearing away of the protective cartilage between bones.

Once this protection is gone, bone can rub on bone. In response, your body may try to generate new bone to replace the lost cartilage. This extra bone, known as a bone spur, usually doesn't cause any signs or symptoms. You may not even realize you have a bone spur until it shows up on an X-ray for another condition. But sometimes the extra bone can narrow the circular space (spinal canal) that spinal nerves pass through. When this happens, the spinal cord or spinal nerve roots may become pinched, causing:

- Pain in your arm and neck
- Numbness or weakness in your arm or forearm
- Tingling in your fingers or hand

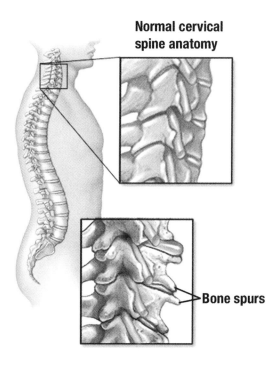

Normal cervical spine anatomy

Bone spurs

Bone spurs. These bony projections can develop along bone edges, including the bones of the spine, and can press on adjacent nerves.

Treatment for a bone spur often includes pain medication and exercises to improve flexibility, strength and posture in hopes of relieving nerve pressure.

Facet joint disease

Facets are the areas where one vertebra connects to another. The connection points between the vertebrae are referred to as the facet joints. These joints provide flexibility, allowing the spine to turn or bend with movement, and stability, preventing excessive motion.

Due to the constant motion of the facet joints, the cartilage that covers the ends of the joints can wear out and become thin, contributing to the growth of bone spurs and enlargement of the joints.

Your risk of facet joint disease increases with age. A history of trauma, degenerative disk disease, poor posture and a family history of degenerative arthritis are other risk factors for the disorder.

Signs and symptoms of facet joint disease include:
- Dull pain and stiffness
- Pain that radiates toward the back of the head, ear or shoulder
- Pain that worsens with movement after a period of inactivity or sleep
- Headaches

Medications to relieve pain and inflammation may be used to treat facet joint disease. Applying heat or ice to the painful area may reduce symptoms. Exercise and physical therapy to correct posture and strengthen muscles also may be recommended. If these steps aren't successful, more-extensive procedures may be necessary.

NERVE-RELATED CONDITIONS

Your spine serves as the main passageway for your spinal cord and other nerves within your nervous system. The spinal cord is a

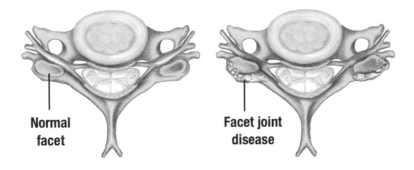

Normal facet

Facet joint disease

Facet joint disease. This spinal condition occurs when the facet joints in the spine degenerate and become inflamed, causing painful symptoms.

ropelike column of nerves that links your brain to the nerves in your arms, legs and trunk. It's surrounded by the small bones (vertebrae) that compose your spinal column, which help protect the cord.

Your cervical spine also contains eight nerve roots that branch out from your neck and help control the function of your shoulders, arms and hands. If your spinal cord or one of these roots becomes compressed or damaged, pain can occur.

Pinched or damaged nerve

Sometimes, neck pain may be traced to a compressed or irritated nerve in the neck, resulting from another condition — such as a herniated disk, spinal stenosis or a bone spur. Rarely, a tumor or an infection can cause nerve damage.

The medical term for radiating pain due to a pinched or damaged nerve is radiculitis. Ra-

diating nerve pain accompanied by neurological symptoms such as numbness or weakness is called radiculopathy. Cervical radiculopathy is the medical term for a range of conditions associated with a pinched or damaged nerve in your neck.

Nerve pain may come on suddenly or more gradually. Depending on what's triggering the pain, it may be a dull ache or a sharp, shooting pain.

You're more likely to develop cervical radiculopathy if you've experienced trauma to your neck or a spinal nerve injury. You may also be at increased risk if your job requires a lot of lifting or you operate heavy equipment that vibrates.

Signs and symptoms of cervical radiculopathy include:
• Neck pain
• Pain in the shoulder blade area
• Arm or hand pain
• Muscle spasms

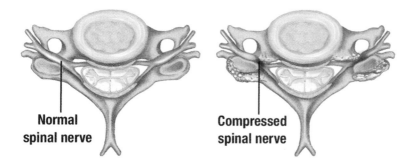

Normal spinal nerve   **Compressed spinal nerve**

Pinched (compressed) nerve. A pinched nerve occurs when too much pressure is applied to a nerve by bone or surrounding tissues, cartilage, muscles or tendons. This pressure disrupts the nerve's function, causing pain, tingling, numbness or weakness.

- Numbness or tingling
- Weakness and lack of coordination in affected arm
- Loss of reflexes

Some people experience relief of their pain when they place the hand of the affected arm on top of their heads. That's because this position may temporarily relieve pressure on the nerve root.

Treatment for cervical radiculopathy includes pain medication, applying heat to the painful area and massage. Depending on the cause, physical therapy also may help alleviate the pain. Injections of medication into the affected nerve (nerve block) also may be used to treat the pain. Only rarely is surgery required.

Accurately diagnosing cervical radiculopathy is important because left untreated the condition can progress to cervical myelopathy, a more serious disorder that can result in paralysis.

Spinal stenosis

Spinal stenosis is the medical term for a narrowing of the space within the spinal canal, resulting in pressure being placed on the nerves that travel through the canal. Spinal stenosis occurs most often in the lower back and the neck. When spinal stenosis occurs in your neck, it's known as cervical stenosis.

Most often, cervical stenosis is brought on by age. Over time, the disks in your spine can dry out and shrink, bringing bones closer together. At the same time, bones and ligaments in the spine can thicken. These factors lead to narrowing of the spinal canal. Stenosis may also result from a bone spur that narrows the spinal canal and presses on spinal nerves.

When pressure is placed on the spinal cord, in addition to your neck, shoulders and arms, you also may experience symptoms in your lower extremities, especially if the

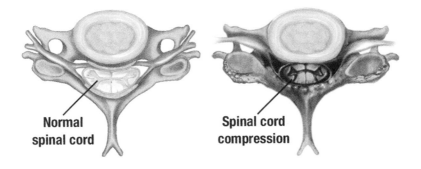

Normal spinal cord

Spinal cord compression

Spinal stenosis. This condition occurs when the space within the spinal canal or around nerve roots becomes narrowed, placing pressure on spinal nerves that travel through the canal, including the spinal cord. Spinal stenosis that occurs in the neck is called cervical stenosis.

compression is more severe. Severe compression is known as cervical myelopathy.

Signs and symptoms of spinal cord compression include:
- Gradual onset of neck pain and stiffness
- Numbness or tingling in a hand or arm, or a foot or leg
- Weakness in a hand or arm, or foot or leg
- Clumsy hands or loss of fine motor skills, such as writing and buttoning clothes
- Problems with balance and walking
- Bowel or bladder dysfunction

Cervical myelopathy can be a medical emergency and may require urgent evaluation. Mild cases may be treated with physical therapy and regular neurological examinations to watch for changes in the condition. More-severe cases or those that are progressing rapidly require surgery to create additional space within the spinal canal, relieving pressure on the spinal cord. Left untreated, the condition can progress to permanent nerve damage and even paralysis.

MALALIGNMENT AND INSTABILITY

Malalignment of the cervical spine refers to a dislocation or change in the position of a joint in the spine — typically slippage of one vertebra onto another. Malalignment can result from several causes, including neck ligaments that become lax, bone degeneration, a fracture or an inflammatory disease, such as rheumatoid arthritis, that damages a cervical joint. Subluxation and spondylolisthesis are medical terms for cervical malalignment.

When a joint isn't aligned properly, pressure may be placed on a spinal nerve. Or the misaligned joint may cause another condition that affects the spinal nerves. Malalignment can produce instability.

Your body has an elaborate system of spinal muscles, tendons and nerves, which adjust to changing spinal loads and help keep your spine stabilized. Nerves attached to your spinal muscles are continuously

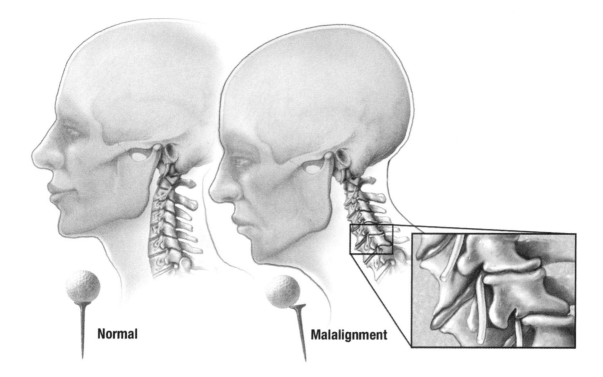

Malalignment. Malalignment refers to a dislocation or change in position of a spinal joint that causes the neck to tilt forward and the cervical spine to become unstable.

transmitting and receiving information about the position of your vertebrae and movement of your body, to inform the muscles what they need to do to help keep your spine stable.

When this control system is unable to compensate for changes in position and weight on the spinal vertebrae — typically due to degenerative conditions or an injury — the spine becomes unstable. This instability can cause structural changes or injury to bone or ligaments, resulting in pain, nerve problems or deformity.

Signs and symptoms of malalignment and instability depend on the specific vertebrae affected. They include:

- Pain that radiates to the back of the head
- Limited motion in the neck due to pain and muscle spasms
- Numbness or loss of sensation in the head
- Difficulties keeping the head up
- Abnormal neck movements, such as accelerated or decelerated movements
- Shakiness or lack of neck control

If malalignment of your cervical spine causes compression of the arteries in your neck, symptoms may develop in your hands and legs, such as numbness, clumsiness, weakness or balance issues. Because this can be life-threatening, it's important to seek medical help if you're experiencing any of these symptoms.

Surgery is generally necessary to treat cervical malalignment and instability and avoid potentially serious complications.

TRAUMA AND FRACTURES

It's important to fully evaluate an injury or accident that causes trauma to your neck. Neck trauma carries the added risk of spinal cord injury and paralysis. Common causes of neck injury are car accidents, diving accidents, sports injuries and falls. An injury also can result in a bone fracture.

Whiplash

A common neck injury is whiplash, which results from forceful, rapid back-and-forth movement of the neck, similar to the cracking of a whip.

Whiplash most often occurs during a rear-end auto accident, when your head is forcefully and quickly thrown backward and then forward. This motion can injure bones in the spine, disks between the bones, ligaments, muscles, nerves and other tissues of the neck. Whiplash also can result from a sports accident, physical abuse or other trauma.

Signs and symptoms of whiplash usually, but not always, develop within 24 hours of the injury. They range from mild to serious and include:
- Neck pain and stiffness
- Worsening of pain with neck movement
- Loss of range of motion in the neck
- Headaches, most often starting at the base of the skull
- Tenderness or pain in the shoulder, upper back or arms
- Tingling or numbness in the arms
- Fatigue
- Dizziness

Some people also experience blurred vision, ringing in the ears (tinnitus), sleep difficulties, concentration difficulties, and mood and memory issues.

Most people get better within a few weeks by following a treatment plan that includes pain medication and exercise. However, some individuals may develop chronic neck pain and headaches that can last for months or years.

Osteoporotic fracture

Bone is living tissue that's constantly being broken down and replaced. Osteoporosis results when the creation of new bone doesn't keep up with the loss of old bone. The disease causes bones to become weak and brittle so that they fracture easily. In addition to a fall, even mild stresses such as bending over or coughing can produce a fracture.

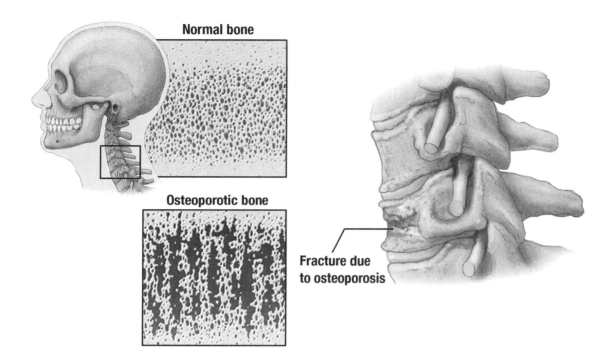

Normal bone

Osteoporotic bone

Fracture due to osteoporosis

Osteoporosis fracture. Weakened bone due to osteoporosis can produce a fracture in a cervical vertebra, causing pain and other symptoms.

Osteoporosis-related cervical fractures are common. In some people, the bones (vertebrae) in the neck can weaken to the point of crumpling, resulting in loss of height and a hunched-forward posture, in addition to pain. Osteoporosis affects men and women of all races, but white and Asian women, especially women past menopause, are at highest risk.

In its early stages, osteoporosis typically doesn't produce any symptoms and people are often unaware of the condition. However, later on, once bones have been weakened, signs and symptoms begin to emerge.

Treatment of osteoporosis generally involves medications, a healthy diet, and weight-bearing exercise aimed at strengthening weakened bone and preventing further bone loss.

Traumatic fracture

On occasion, an accident or injury can cause a bone in the neck to fracture. This is known as a cervical fracture, which is sometimes referred to as a "broken neck." This type of injury usually results from some type of violent trauma, such as a car crash, a fall or contact while playing sports. A cervical fracture is very serious. In some cases, it can result in paralysis from the neck down and even death.

Signs and symptoms of a neck fracture include:
- Temporary or permanent paralysis
- Severe neck pain, which may spread down to the shoulders or arms
- Bruising and swelling of the neck

If a neck fracture is suspected, it's best not to move the individual and to wait for emergency help to arrive. Emergency responders will immobilize the neck to protect it against further damage until X-rays can be done to assess the situation.

Treatment for a neck fracture depends on which vertebra suffered the damage and the type of fracture. Minor compression fractures may require wearing a neck brace for several weeks while the bone heals. More-severe fractures may require a combination of treatments, including traction, surgery and use of a neck cast.

Spinal cord injury

Approximately 300,000 people in the United States live with a spinal cord injury. A spinal cord injury occurs when any part of the spinal cord or the nerves at the end of the spinal canal (cauda equina) are damaged. Spinal cord injury often causes permanent changes in strength, sensation and other body functions below the site of the injury.

Scientists are hopeful that advances in research will someday make the repair of spinal cord injuries possible. Research studies are ongoing around the world. In the meantime, medical treatments and rehabilitation therapy allow many people with spinal cord injuries to lead productive, independent lives.

Symptoms Spinal cord injuries of any kind may result in one or more of the following signs and symptoms. The degree to which these signs and symptoms affect an individual depends on the level and completeness of the injury.
- Loss of strength
- Loss of or altered sensation, including the ability to feel heat, cold and touch
- Loss of bowel or bladder control
- Exaggerated reflex activities or spasms
- Changes in sexual function, sexual sensitivity and fertility
- Pain or an intense stinging sensation caused by damage to the nerve fibers in your spinal cord
- Difficulty breathing, coughing or clearing secretions from your lungs

Causes Spinal cord injury results from damage to the spinal cord itself, due to trauma of structures such as the vertebrae, ligaments or disks of the spinal column, or to nontraumatic causes such as cancer, bleeding and infection.

A traumatic spinal cord injury may stem from a sudden, traumatic blow to your spine that fractures, dislocates, crushes or compresses one or more of your vertebrae.

Spinal cord injuries are most commonly caused by an accident or fall but may also result from a gunshot or knife wound that penetrates and cuts the spinal cord.

The most common causes of spinal cord injuries in the United States are:

- **Motor vehicle accidents.** Auto and motorcycle accidents are the leading cause of spinal cord injuries, accounting for almost half of new spinal cord injuries each year.
- **Falls.** A spinal cord injury after age 65 is most often caused by a fall.
- **Acts of violence.** Some spinal cord injuries result from violent encounters, most commonly involving gunshot wounds. Knife wounds also are common.
- **Sports and recreation injuries.** Athletic activities, such as impact sports and diving in shallow water, cause about 10% of spinal cord injuries.
- **Alcohol.** Alcohol use is a factor in some spinal cord injuries.
- **Disease.** Cancer, arthritis, osteoporosis, and inflammation or infection of the spinal cord can cause spinal cord injuries.

Additional damage usually occurs over days or weeks after the injury because of bleeding, swelling, inflammation and fluid accumulation in and around your spinal cord.

Whether the cause is traumatic or nontraumatic, the damage affects the nerve fibers passing through the injured area and may impair part or all of your corresponding muscles and nerves below the injury site.

A chest (thoracic) or lower back (lumbar) injury can affect your torso, legs, bowel and bladder control, and sexual function. A neck (cervical) injury affects the same areas in addition to affecting movements of your arms and, possibly, your ability to breathe.

An injury to your cervical or thoracic spine may also affect your ability to maintain your blood pressure, body temperature and other bodily functions.

Diagnosis and care Tests used to diagnose a spinal cord injury include X-rays, computerized tomography (CT) scans, and magnetic resonance imaging (MRI).

A few days after injury, when some of the swelling may have subsided, your doctor may conduct a more comprehensive neurological exam to determine the level and completeness of your injury. This involves testing your muscle strength and your ability to sense light touch and pinprick sensations.

Unfortunately, there's no way to reverse damage to the spinal cord. However, scientists and researchers are continually working on new treatments, including prostheses and medications that may promote nerve cell regeneration or improve the function of the nerves that remain after a spinal cord injury.

In the meantime, treatment focuses on preventing further injury and empowering people with a spinal cord injury to return to an active and productive life.

CLASSIFICATIONS

Your ability to control your limbs after a spinal cord injury depends on two factors: the location of the injury along your spinal cord and the severity of injury. The severity of the injury is often called "the completeness" and is classified as either of the following:

- **Complete.** If all feeling (sensory) and all ability to control movement (motor function) are lost below the level of the spinal cord injury, your injury is called complete.
- **Incomplete.** If you have some motor or sensory function below the affected area, your injury is called incomplete. There are varying degrees of incomplete injury.

Additionally, paralysis from a spinal cord injury may be referred to as:

- **Tetraplegia.** Also known as quadriplegia, this means that your arms, hands, trunk, legs and pelvic organs are all affected by your spinal cord injury.
- **Paraplegia.** This paralysis affects all or part of the trunk, legs and pelvic organs.

Rehabilitation Rehabilitation team members begin their work in the early stages of recovery. Your team may include a physical therapist, an occupational therapist, a rehabilitation nurse, a rehabilitation psychologist, a social worker, a dietitian, a recreation therapist, and a doctor who specializes in physical medicine (physiatrist) or spinal cord injuries.

Following surgical or medical treatment that may be needed to help stabilize the spine after a spinal cord injury, the next step generally is intensive inpatient rehabilitation involving a multidisciplinary approach to care.

During the initial stages of rehabilitation, therapists usually emphasize maintenance and strengthening of existing muscle function, redeveloping fine motor skills, and learning adaptive techniques to accomplish day-to-day tasks.

The goal of inpatient rehabilitation is to allow you to develop the tools needed to live as productively and independently as possible.

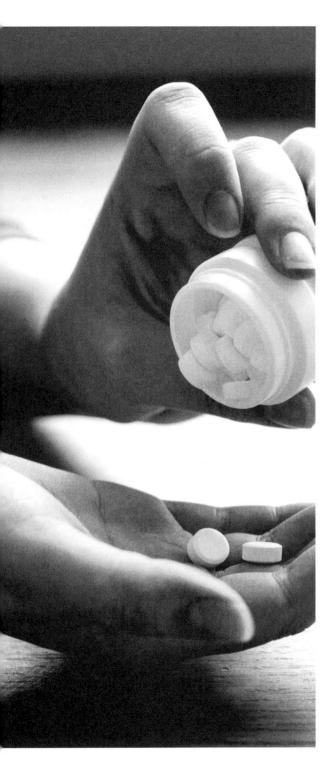

You'll be educated on the effects of a spinal cord injury and how to prevent complications, and you'll be given advice on rebuilding your life and increasing your quality of life and independence. You'll also be taught many new skills, and you'll be introduced to equipment and technologies that can help you live on your own as much as possible. Family members will also receive guidance on how to support you.

Medications Medications may be used to manage some of the effects of spinal cord injury. These include drugs to control pain and muscle spasticity, as well as medications that can improve bladder and bowel control, blood pressure control, and sexual function.

New technologies and treatments Inventive medical devices can help people with a spinal cord injury become more independent and more mobile. Some devices may also help restore motor function. Your medical and therapy teams will help guide you in what types of technologies and treatments might be helpful in your individual case. These include:

- **Electrical stimulation devices.** These sophisticated devices use electrical stimulation to produce muscle activity. They're often called functional electrical stimulation systems, and they use electrical stimulators to activate arm and leg muscles to allow people with spinal cord injuries to stand, walk, reach and grip.
- **Robotic gait training.** This emerging technology is used to help regain the ability to walk after a spinal cord injury.

- **Stem cell therapy.** Stem cell therapy is a rapidly evolving treatment for spinal cord injuries. Stem cells are self-renewing human cells that can evolve into one or more specific cell types. Successful stem cell treatment may limit existing neuronal cell death, stimulate growth from existing cells, and replace injured cells, facilitating movement. It is important to remember, however, that stem cell therapies are still experimental and more research is needed to demonstrate their safety and effectiveness.

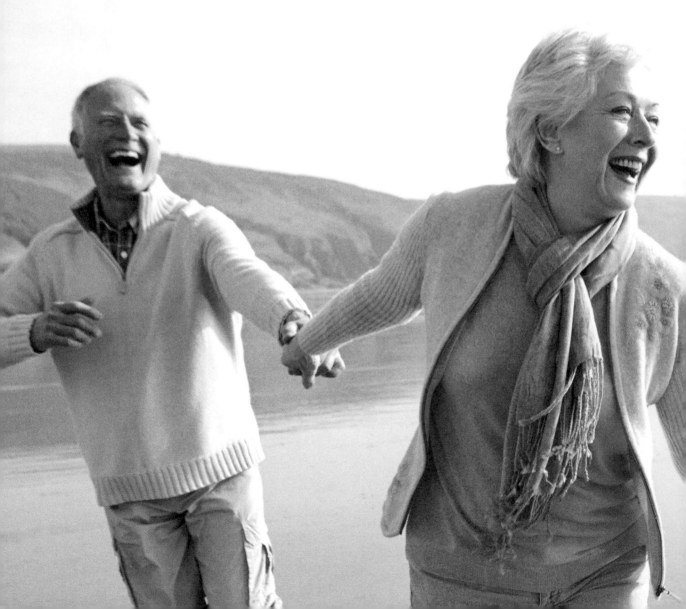

Relieving your pain

CHAPTER 5

Identifying the problem

In the first part of this book, you learned how your back and neck work, and you got a glimpse into common back and neck conditions. In part 2, we'll focus on finding relief for your pain.

Knowing that neck and back pain are familiar experiences for many people doesn't necessarily make it any easier when you're dealing with your own symptoms. Conditions that affect your back and neck can be painful and disruptive. But it's important that you not ignore back and neck pain if the pain is severe or it persists for more than a few weeks. Pain is your body's way of warning you that something is wrong.

Back and neck conditions can occur for a variety of reasons. To effectively treat the accompanying pain, it's helpful to know the cause — where the pain is originating.

Sometimes this can be easy to determine; other times it's more difficult. When you meet with your doctor, be aware that you might not get answers right away. Identifying what may be triggering your pain can be a process that takes time to sort out.

If you're worried about your condition, that's understandable. Many people feel stressed and afraid because they don't know what's happening, and the unknown can be scary. Having an idea of what to expect when you see a medical provider may reduce your anxiety and make the experience seem less stressful.

DESCRIBING YOUR PAIN

Pain is an individual experience, and some people find it difficult to talk about being in pain. But if you want relief, it's important that you be open and honest with your doctor about what you're feeling. Being in pain isn't a sign of weakness, nor does it indicate that you can't handle your condition.

Common questions

Expect your doctor to ask you a number of questions about your pain. He or she will want to know about what you're feeling and how it's affecting you.

When did the pain begin? This question isn't merely about the time and date you began hurting. Your doctor may ask:

- Were you injured or in an accident? If so, how and when?
- Did your pain begin abruptly or develop over time?
- Have you had previous episodes? If so, when and how does your current pain compare?
- Has your pain worsened or stayed the same since it began?

Where does it hurt? The site of your pain can provide insight into a possible cause. Sometimes pain is limited to a specific area. In other cases, it can extend to other body parts. For example, back pain may spread into the buttocks, outer hip, down a leg or even into a foot.

What does it feel like? Describe how your pain feels. The type of pain you're experiencing may help determine the underlying cause.

Descriptions commonly used to describe pain include sharp and stabbing, dull and achy, or burning. Some people describe a "charley-horse" type of cramp or spasm, or you may have a burning sensation in your lower back. Your pain may be constant throughout the day or it may come and go and develop with certain activities, movements or positions.

It's also not uncommon for pain to be accompanied by other sensations. You may experience numbness or tingling that may be confined to your neck or back or spread to your arms and legs. You may notice weakness that affects your ability to move or complete tasks.

How much does it hurt? There are several ways to gauge your pain level. You may be asked whether your pain is mild, moderate or severe. Sometimes doctors use a pain scale, which asks you to measure your pain on a zero to 10 scale, with zero being no pain and 10 being the worst pain you can imagine. Another common way doctors measure pain is by showing you pictures of faces with different expressions of discomfort and asking you to choose the one that most closely resembles how you feel.

In addition to rating your pain, explain to your doctor how your pain has affected your daily routine. Discuss any changes in your sleep habits and quality of sleep. If your condition has affected your ability to do your job, perform routine tasks at home, or spend time with family and friends, mention this as well. Also, don't be afraid to let

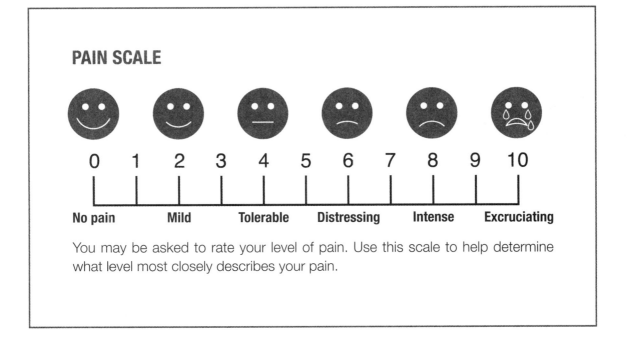

PAIN SCALE

0 1 2 3 4 5 6 7 8 9 10

No pain   Mild   Tolerable   Distressing   Intense   Excruciating

You may be asked to rate your level of pain. Use this scale to help determine what level most closely describes your pain.

your doctor know how you're feeling emotionally.

When and how often does it hurt? Pain can be constant, or it can come and go throughout the day. It's not unusual to feel stiffness and soreness in the morning that lessens throughout the day. Or it may be that your pain builds throughout the day and is worse in the evening or at night.

Also, is there anything you do that makes your pain worse? Is it affected by certain movements or activities? This may include activities such as lifting, bending, resting, sitting, standing or reclining.

If there are things you do that seem to lessen your pain, be sure to let your doctor know. Does changing positions help you feel better? Does your pain improve when you stand and walk or when you sit down or lie flat? If you've tried heating pads or ice packs, how did it go? Did they alleviate your pain? Have you tried pain medications? If so, did they help? Have you had any tests done for your current condition or a similar disorder? What were the results?

A PHYSICAL EXAM

Once your medical provider is done asking questions, he or she will likely want to do a physical examination. In addition to helping to make a diagnosis, an exam can help determine if further testing may be needed.

Your exam may begin with an inspection of your neck and back and your posture while standing and sitting. By observing your spine while you stand, your doctor can evaluate the alignment of your spine and observe any structural issues, such as an abnormal curvature.

Your doctor may feel (palpate) areas along your neck and back in an attempt to locate sources of pain, tenderness or spasm.

He or she may also check your range of motion to identify any limitations that may point to a specific issue, such as a joint problem, muscle sprain or a nerve disorder. You may be asked to:

- Move your neck side to side as well as forward and backward and in a twisting motion
- Bend in a forward, backward, twisting and side-to-side motion at the waist
- Walk across the room
- Raise a leg straight out in front of you

Your exam may also include a check of your neurological function. Your spine protects many of your body's nerves, including the spinal cord and spinal nerves. In search of the source of your pain, your doctor may try to evaluate how your nerves are working. He or she may observe your gait while walking, test your reflexes and muscle strength, and determine if you can identify different sensations such as touch, sharpness and temperature.

Results from your physical exam may provide clues as to where the pain may be coming from and help rule out more-serious causes of spine pain.

Based on what he or she has learned, your doctor will decide if further tests are needed. If there's reason to suspect that a specific condition is causing your pain, your doctor might order one or more tests. A variety of tests may be used to provide information about what's happening within the structures of your back and neck.

IMAGING TESTS

Several imaging tests may be used to help diagnose back and neck conditions. The type of test you have will likely be determined by your symptoms, your doctor's preferences, your insurance and the availability of the tests.

X-ray

An X-ray (radiograph) is a safe, quick and painless test that produces images of the structures inside your body, chiefly your bones.

How it works X-ray beams pass through your body and are absorbed in different amounts depending on the density of the material they pass through. Dense bone absorbs much of the X-ray radiation, while soft tissues, such as muscles, fat and organs, allow more of the radiation to pass through them. As a result, your bones appear white on the pictures, soft tissue shows up in shades of gray and air is black.

X-rays of the neck or back are usually done while you're standing. This allows your doctor to view your back while it's bearing your body's weight. You may be given a lead apron to place over your breasts or pelvic area to protect those areas from radiation. Several images are taken from different directions and sometimes while you're bending forward or backward.

You'll be asked to hold still and perhaps hold your breath while the images are taken. An individual X-ray usually takes just a moment, and the entire series of images is often obtained in only five to 10 minutes.

Uses An X-ray can help diagnose the following problems that may be linked to neck or back pain:
- **Fracture.** In most cases, an X-ray can detect a fractured bone. Subsequent X-rays can help monitor how well the fracture is healing.
- **Arthritis.** An X-ray of your joints can reveal signs of arthritis.
- **Bone issues.** An X-ray can identify an injury, infection, bone growth and bony changes.
- **Cancer.** An X-ray can reveal a tumor that may be cancerous.

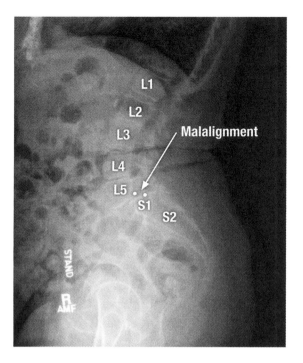

This X-ray, a side view of the lumbar spine, indicates malalignment of the spine between vertebrae L5 and S1 (see arrow). Vertebra L5 has shifted forward and no longer sits directly above vertebra S1. Adjoining bone segments (indicated by the two dots) should line up to maintain the gradual S curve. Note: Each vertebra in your spine is assigned a letter correlating with the region of the spine where it is located — C, T, L or S — and a number.

Benefits X-rays are commonly taken because they're noninvasive, painless, relatively inexpensive and they generally don't cause side effects. However, plain X-rays alone often aren't enough to diagnose a spinal condition. Other tests are needed to confirm a diagnosis.

Risks Because radiation is used, having an X-ray may slightly increase your risk of developing cancer later in life. However, the risk is extremely small, and the benefit of an accurate diagnosis far outweighs the risk. Special care is taken during an X-ray to deliver the least amount of radiation while still getting the best possible image. X-rays shouldn't be used if there's a possibility that you're pregnant. If you're pregnant or think you might be, be sure to tell your doctor.

Limitations An X-ray provides detailed pictures of your bones, but it doesn't offer much information about your muscles, tendons, joints or disks. Another imaging test, such as an MRI or CT scan, is needed to gather information on those structures.

Computerized tomography (CT) scan

A CT scan uses X-ray technology, but instead of a single flat image, it produces multiple cross-sectional images. The images show details of not only your bones but also your organs, blood, blood vessels and soft tissues, including the disks between the vertebrae in your spine and some of the soft tissue of the spinal cord. Like an X-ray, a CT is painless and noninvasive.

How it works A CT scan follows much the same principle as an X-ray. While an X-ray examines one part of your body to develop a single picture, a CT scan combines a series of X-ray images taken from different angles with computer processing to create cross-sectional images of your body. This allows your doctor to see inside the structures of your back and neck from different viewpoints, including front to back, side to side and top to bottom. A CT scan can even make 3D images of a particular part of your body.

For the exam, you lie flat on your back on a motorized table. Pillows and straps may help you remain in still. During the scan, the table will move through the scanner, which is shaped like a large doughnut standing on its side. The scanner will rotate around you as it creates the images. You may hear buzzing and whirring noises as the table moves during the scan. A CT scan is usually completed within 30 minutes. Much of that time is preparation work with only about 10 minutes spent on the imaging table.

Uses A CT scan is used most often to determine if there's been damage to the spinal column. The images it provides can help your doctor:

- Distinguish between bone and soft tissue to find the source of your pain
- Diagnose diseases and disorders of the muscle, soft tissues and bone, such as bone tumors and fractures
- Pinpoint the location of a tumor, infection or blood clot
- Detect spinal abnormalities, such as a curvature of the spine
- Help perform a diagnostic procedure, such as a biopsy of a suspicious area to detect cancer or to remove fluid from an infected area

- Measure bone density in your spine to help predict your risk of vertebral fractures if you have osteoporosis

If you have spinal stenosis, a condition that causes narrowing of the spinal canal, or a fractured vertebrae or arthritis, CT scans of your spine can provide valuable information to help manage and treat those conditions.

Benefits The test is quick, painless and non-invasive. It's less sensitive to movements than magnetic resonance imaging (MRI), and unlike an MRI, it can be performed even if you have an implanted medical device or metal in your body. There are no immediate side effects, and no radiation remains in your body after the exam.

Risks During the test, you're briefly exposed to ionizing radiation. The amount of radiation is greater than that of an X-ray because more pictures are taken. The radiation hasn't been shown to cause long-term harm, but there may be a very small increase in your potential risk of cancer. However, the benefits that can come from a detailed look at your neck and back exceed any potential risks of the test. If there's a possibility that you're pregnant, make sure to tell your doctor.

Limitations A very large person may not fit into the opening of a conventional CT scanner. There is also a weight limit for the moving table. A CT scan of the spine may not provide enough detail of the spinal cord, disks and other soft tissues. In addition, if you've had hardware, such as rods and screws, placed in your spine during previous surgeries, the images likely will be affected.

Magnetic resonance imaging (MRI)

Magnetic resonance imaging uses a magnetic field and radio waves to create detailed images of the organs and tissues within your body. An MRI machine creates images of your spine and its surrounding structures, including adjacent nerves and tissues, from different angles. The procedure is painless and noninvasive.

How it works Unlike an X-ray or CT scan, an MRI doesn't involve radiation. Instead, the machine creates a temporary magnetic field around your body, which realigns the water molecules inside your body. Radio waves cause the realigned atoms to produce very faint signals. A computer converts the signals into cross-sectional or 3D images that may be viewed from many different angles.

An MRI machine looks like a long narrow tube that's open on both ends. It's narrower and longer than a CT machine. You lie on a movable table that slides into the tube. Because any movement can blur the pictures, pillows, props and straps may be used to help you hold still. While you don't feel the magnetic field or the radio waves, the magnets can make loud noises, so you'll likely be given earplugs.

There isn't a lot of space inside an MRI machine, and this is an issue for some people. There are some types of scanners in which the magnets don't completely surround you or the opening is larger in diameter. While an open MRI may feel more comfortable, it can take longer to get the images, and the images produced may not be optimal. An MRI can last anywhere from 15 minutes to more than an hour.

Uses MRI images of your back or neck can help your doctor:
- Examine the anatomy and alignment of your spine
- Detect injury to bones, disks, ligaments or your spinal cord
- Diagnose disk and joint disease
- Identify compression or inflammation of the spinal cord and spinal nerves
- Identify an infection of a vertebra, disk, spinal cord or its coverings (meninges)
- Locate tumors in the spinal cord, vertebrae, nerves or surrounding soft tissues
- Detect a compression fracture and bone swelling
- Identify birth defects in the vertebrae or spinal cord

Your doctor may also use an MRI to guide treatment. For example, if you're diagnosed with a pinched nerve, he or she will use MRI images to help identify the location and cause. MRI images may also be used to guide steroid injections to make sure the medication is placed in the right location. After surgery, if an individual isn't improving, an MRI may be repeated to determine why the person isn't responding.

Benefits MRIs can produce images of any part of your body from any direction. They

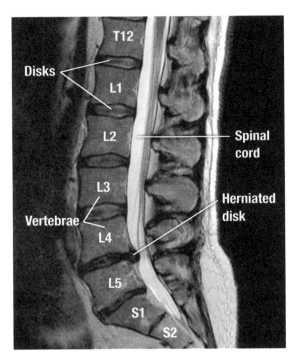

MRI scan A side view of the lumbar spine is shown in this MRI scan. The scan reveals a herniated disk between vertebrae L4 and L5 (see the arrow). The ruptured disk is pressing on adjacent spinal nerves.

provide clearer, more-detailed images of soft tissues than does a CT scan. A CT is usually better at imaging bones, while an MRI can better differentiate between fat, water, muscle and other soft tissues.

An MRI is the best test for visualizing the spinal cord and nerves and evaluating ligament injuries. An MRI is also better at identifying tumors and other masses near the spinal cord, and it can detect abnormalities that might be obscured by bone on a CT.

Risks The magnetic field created by an MRI isn't harmful, but it may interfere with medical devices or pieces of metal in your body. The machine's magnetic force can cause the implants or metal to heat up and move, causing potential harm or distorting the images. For this reason, you'll likely be asked to complete a questionnaire before the procedure about any electronic devices or metal in your body.

There are no known risks when safety guidelines are followed. The procedure can trigger feelings of claustrophobia in some individuals, who may require sedation. While there's no reason to believe that an MRI can harm a fetus, tell your doctor if there's a possibility that you're pregnant.

Limitations Image quality depends on your ability to remain still and follow breath-holding instructions while the images are being recorded. If you're anxious, confused or in pain, you may find it difficult to lie still. Some imaging centers may give you a mild sedating medication if you meet the criteria to receive the medication and you have someone to drive you home. There also are weight limits on scanners, and a person who is very large may not fit into some MRI machines.

Because most MRI scans are performed while you're lying down, the test doesn't show what the spine looks like when you're standing and bearing weight. In addition, an MRI typically costs more and takes more time to perform than other medical imaging techniques.

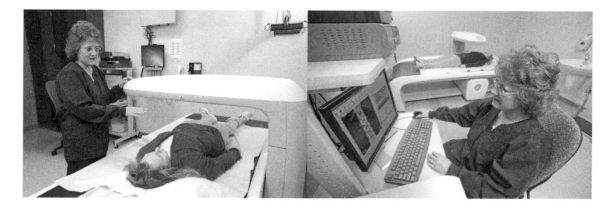

Bone density test These photos show a dual-energy X-ray absorptiometry (DXA or DEXA) scan of the spine. For this test, you lie flat on your back and the arm of the device is positioned over your spine. The arm measures your bone density by detecting energy from an X-ray source located under the table. The information is transmitted to a computer, where an image of your spine appears, along with a summary of your bone density measurements.

Bone density test

If your doctor suspects that your back or neck symptoms may be related to osteoporosis, he or she recommend a bone density test. Osteoporosis causes your bones to become fragile, making them more likely to fracture. The bones of the lower back are especially susceptible to fracture among people with osteoporosis.

If you've lost height, have unexplained back pain or have a vertebral fracture that occurred more easily than expected, you may need a bone density test to determine if you have osteoporosis or are at risk. Bones most commonly tested include the spine and hips.

With this test, X-rays pass through your body and measure how many grams of cal-

cium and other minerals are contained in a segment of bone. The results estimate your bone's strength and the likelihood of it breaking. The test is painless and noninvasive, and it usually takes about 10 to 30 minutes. Let your doctor know if there's a possibility that you're pregnant. During the test, part of your body is exposed to a small dose of radiation.

ENHANCED IMAGING TESTS

Sometimes an imaging test may include use of a contrast material — called a contrast agent, medium or dye — to help distinguish certain areas of your body from surrounding tissues. A contrast material can enhance images of your neck and back to help identify possible sources of your pain.

The contrast is generally placed into your body through a vein in your arm before the exam begins. The agent may be iodine-based (for CT images) or contain a material called gadolinium (for MRI testing). Contrast materials, which are safe to use in most instances, temporarily change the way imaging tools interact with the body. They don't discolor the inside of your body.

Following the exam, the material is safely eliminated by your body. Adverse reactions are uncommon, and serious allergic reactions are rare. Risk of a serious reaction to gadolinium is increased if you have kidney problems, so be sure to tell your doctor if you have impaired renal function.

The following tests involve the use a contrast material.

Myelography

Myelography uses contrast material to look at the spinal cord, nerve roots and meninges, the coverings that surround the spinal cord and nerve roots.

How it works During this test you're positioned on your abdomen or side while contrast material is injected into the space around your spinal cord and nerve roots. For the test, you lie on your abdomen. The exam table is slowly tilted, allowing the contrast material to flow up or down through the spaces in the spinal canal. Real-time images of your spine are captured and viewed by a doctor.

You may be repositioned throughout the procedure to get more images. Your doctor may also want a CT scan performed afterward, while the contrast material is still present in your spinal canal. The procedure usually takes 30 to 60 minutes to complete.

Uses A myelogram is an effective alternative for people who can't have an MRI. It can identify many of the same conditions as an MRI, including compression of the spinal cord or spinal nerves or narrowing of the spinal canal, as well as detect tumors, infection, disease and trauma. Tell your doctor if you're pregnant or breast-feeding.

Benefits Myelography is relatively safe and painless. It allows your doctor to see areas on the spine that aren't visible on X-rays.

Risks The main disadvantage of the procedure is that it's invasive, requiring use of a needle. Rare complications include bleeding, inflammation and infection around the nerve roots or spinal membranes. Seizure is a very rare complication.

Although uncommon, there's a risk of a headache, which may occur two to three days following the exam. The headache usually develops when you sit or stand and it improves when you lie down. If the headache is severe, contact your doctor. If the headache persists, your doctor may do a simple procedure called an epidural blood patch to help relieve it.

Limitations Myelography only offers views inside the spinal canal and around the spinal nerve roots. An MRI or CT may be better at revealing problems outside these areas.

Bone scan

For unexplained bone pain, a bone scan (radionuclide bone scan) can help diagnose a variety of bone diseases and conditions, including fractures, infection and cancer.

The procedure involves a radioactive tracer that's placed in a vein in an arm. Areas of the body where cells and tissues are repairing themselves take up the largest amounts of the tracer. These areas are detected with a special camera.

The test takes two to four hours, to allow time for the radiotracer to circulate through your body before the imaging is done. The test uses less radiation than a CT scan, and the tracer will pass out of your body through urine or stool within a few hours or days following the test. Let your doctor know if you're pregnant or breast-feeding.

Discography

This procedure is rarely used today. For the test, a contrast material is injected into a protruding disk to determine if the disk may be causing low back pain. Discography can result in increased pain and rarely infection and it can produce false positives, indicating a disk is at fault when it's really not. Additional complications may include headaches, nausea, blood vessel or nerve

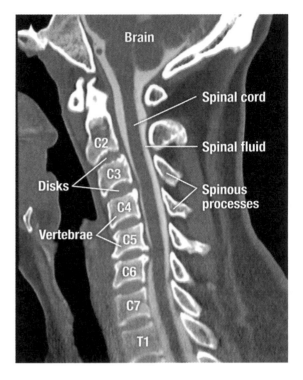

CT myelogram This CT myelogram image shows a side view of a neck (cervical spine). A CT scan provides more detailed bone anatomy images than does an X-ray. The contrast material used in the procedure makes the spinal cord and spinal fluid more visual.

injury, bleeding, and temporary numbness or weakness. There's a very small risk of paralysis.

BEYOND IMAGING

Other tests may be performed occasionally to help determine the cause of neck and back pain.

OTHER CONDITIONS THAT CAN CAUSE BACK PAIN

Sometimes, back or neck pain has nothing to do with your back or neck! The pain may originate in other areas of your body and radiate to your spine or pelvis. Diagnostic tests can help determine if the culprit of your discomfort is your back or neck or if the pain is associated with a condition elsewhere in your body.

Some conditions that may cause back and neck pain include:
- **Kidney stones or infections.** The pain is usually on one side of the lower back.
- **Endometriosis.** Pain with this disorder may spread beyond the female pelvic organs to the back.
- **Fibromyalgia.** It causes widespread muscle pain and fatigue, including the back and neck.
- **Shoulder conditions.** Injury in the shoulder, such as a torn rotator cuff or shoulder impingement, may cause neck pain.
- **Cardiovascular conditions.** An abdominal aortic aneurysm, tear in a major blood vessel, or a heart condition can mimic neck or back pain.

Nerve studies

For symptoms such as numbness, tingling, weakness, muscle cramping or certain types of limb pain, a test called an electromyogram (EMG) may be used.

This test is performed to assess the health of muscles and nerve cells (motor neurons) that control muscles. Motor neurons transmit electrical signals that cause your muscles to contract. An EMG test uses tiny electrodes to translate these signals into graphs, sounds or numerical values interpreted by a doctor.

Test results can reveal muscle dysfunction, nerve dysfunction or other problems with nerve-to-muscle transmission.

Two parts For one part of this test, called needle EMG, a thin needle electrode is inserted through the skin and into a muscle, where it records the electrical activity in that muscle. Electrodes may be inserted into various muscles. By studying the electrical signals made during needle EMG, your doctor can evaluate how well your individual muscles and nerves are working. There may be a small amount of pain from the insertion of the needle.

In the second part of the test, called a nerve conduction study, peripheral nerves are stimulated with electricity, and the time it takes to produce motor or sensory messages is measured. Stimulating the electrodes can cause a brief electrical, tingling feeling. The test measures the speed and strength of the signals traveling between two or more points along a nerve to measure nerve communication. Several nerves may be tested.

Uses Nerve study results can help your doctor diagnose or rule out a number of conditions, including:

- Muscle disorders, such as muscular dystrophy or myositis
- Muscle and nerve connection disorders, such as myasthenia gravis
- Disorders affecting motor neurons in the brain or spinal cord, such as amyotrophic lateral sclerosis or spinal muscular atrophy
- Nerve root disorders, such as a pinched nerve or a herniated disk

Blood tests

Most people with a neck or back condition don't require blood testing. However, blood tests may be helpful if your doctor suspects that your pain might be caused by an infection, inflammation or cancer. In particular, your doctor may look at your erythrocyte sedimentation rate (ESR), C-reactive protein (CRP) or both.

An ESR test measures the distance red blood cells fall in a tiny capillary tube in one hour.

The farther the red blood cells fall, the greater your immune system's inflammatory response. The test can help indicate if your symptoms may stem from an inflammatory disorder, such as giant cell arteritis, polymyalgia rheumatica or rheumatoid arthritis.

CRP also measures inflammation. In addition to infection, increased CRP levels may indicate a chronic noninfectious inflammatory disease or even heart disease.

GETTING A SECOND OPINION

Dealing with a complicated medical condition can feel overwhelming at times, and it's normal to have questions and concerns. Seeking a second or even third opinion is a reasonable approach if doing so will help you feel more confident about the diagnosis you've been given and plans for treatment.

There are many reasons why you may want to seek another opinion. Maybe your provider isn't an expert in your condition or he or she is having trouble making a diagnosis. Maybe your current treatment plan isn't working. Perhaps you're having difficulty understanding your condition and you'd like the condition and options for treatment explained by someone else. Also, because doctors often have areas of specialty, your doctor may prefer an approach to treatment that you don't agree with or feel isn't best for you.

To get a second opinion, you can ask your doctor to refer you to someone else. You can also ask family members or friends who've been treated for similar conditions about their experiences. Another option is to check with your insurance company for a list of approved providers.

If the second opinion results agree with the first, you can feel more confident that you're taking the right approach. If the opinions differ, you'll have to decide which option you feel is best. Consider what issues are most important to you and what you feel makes the most sense. If you're having difficulty making a decision, seek out a medical provider who knows you and whom you trust, such as your family physician. Ask him or her to review the information with you and help you reach a decision.

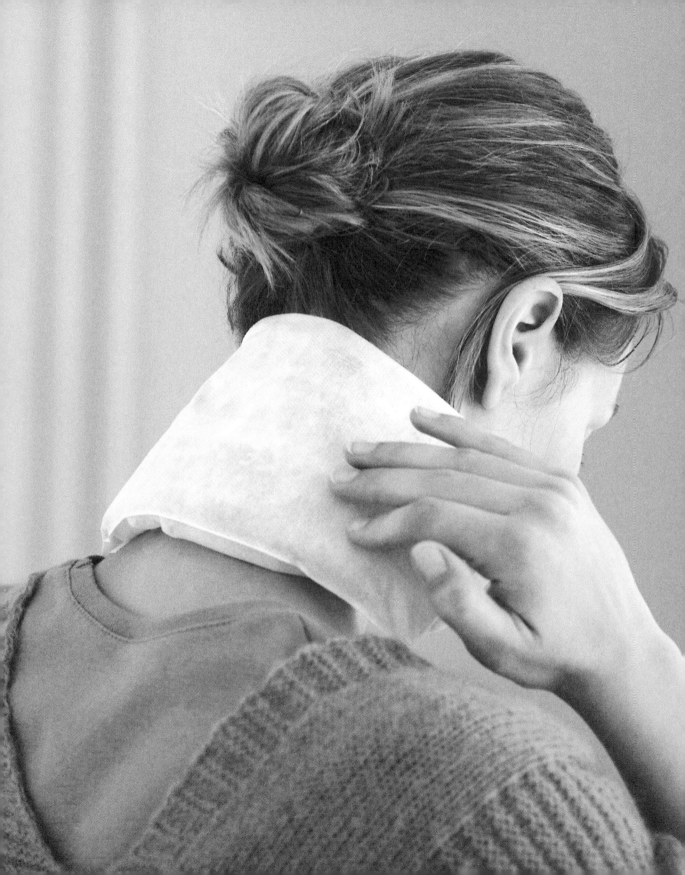

CHAPTER 6

Home treatment

Back and neck pain can strike when you least expect it. Your first tennis match in months leaves your lower back aching. A night sleeping in an awkward position results in a stiff, sore neck. One wrong twist while weeding your flowers sends a stab of pain through your back or neck that doesn't go away.

The good news is that most back and neck pain gradually improves within a few days or weeks without a visit to your doctor. Often you can treat the injury or muscle strain on your own with some simple self-care strategies.

This chapter offers suggestions for relieving short-term (acute) back and neck problems at home so that you can return to your normal activities. Many of these remedies may also help improve back or neck pain that lasts for four to 12 weeks (subacute) or more than 12 weeks (chronic) when used in tandem with treatment from your medical provider.

SELF-CARE AT HOME

Most cases of back and neck pain aren't serious and can be managed on their own. It's appropriate to treat back and neck pain at home if your pain:
- Doesn't progressively worsen over time
- Doesn't spread to one or both legs or arms
- Isn't accompanied by weakness, numbness or tingling in your legs or arms, or numbness in your genital area
- Doesn't keep you from walking and generally going about your daily activities
- Gradually improves within three to six weeks

If you have worsening pain or notice a change in signs and symptoms, contact your doctor. In some cases, back or neck pain can be a symptom of a more serious problem. To learn more about when to see a medical provider for neck or back pain, turn to page 33.

HOW TO EASE THE PAIN

There are a number of steps you can take to ease your discomfort and help your body heal. You may find that some options are more helpful than others. Listen to your body and do what's most effective for you.

Hot and cold compression

When you hurt, it's difficult to think about anything other than your pain. You want relief, and you want it fast. Cold, heat or a combination of the two may help. Applying ice to a sore back or the base of the neck can numb the pain and may reduce some inflammation caused by a minor injury, such as a muscle strain.

Try wrapping an ice pack or a bag of frozen vegetables in a cloth and applying it to the painful area. Do this for the first day or two after your injury, every two to four hours. Don't keep the cold wrap on the painful area for more than 20 minutes at a time.

Heat helps relax and loosen tense muscles, which can reduce pain. Use a heating pad or a moist towel warmed in the microwave and apply it to your back or neck. Or you can take a warm bath or shower. Apply the heat for up to 20 minutes three times a day. If you use a heating pad, never sleep with it.

Some people find that heat works best to relieve their pain. Others prefer ice or a combination of heat and ice. You might need to experiment to figure out what is most effective for you.

Over-the-counter pain relievers

Nonprescription pain medications are another way to quickly reduce pain and discomfort. These medications, called analgesics, help control pain by interfering with the development, transmission and interpretation of pain messages.

Nonsteroidal anti-inflammatory drugs (NSAIDs) NSAIDs such as ibuprofen (Advil, Motrin IB, others) and naproxen sodium (Aleve) generally work best for relieving acute low back and neck pain. In addition to controlling pain, they reduce inflammation. Take these medications only in the recommended dose. Overuse can cause side effects, including nausea, stomach pain, or even stomach bleeding and ulcers. Large doses can also lead to kidney problems and high blood pressure.

Acetaminophen If you can't tolerate NSAIDs, acetaminophen (Tylenol, others) may provide some pain relief if your back or neck is hurting. Unlike NSAIDs, acetaminophen doesn't fight inflammation.

When taken as recommended, acetaminophen has a low risk of side effects. Taking higher doses, however, brings an increased risk of liver or kidney damage.

Topical pain relievers Topical pain relievers are creams, gels, sprays and patches that are applied to the skin at the area of pain. Topical pain relievers may help reduce mild to moderate pain without serious side effects — in part because they're applied locally instead of being circulated throughout the body. Follow the directions on the label. Common topical pain relievers include:

- **Capsaicin.** Capsaicin topicals (Capzasin, Zostrix, others) cause the burning sensation you associate with chili peppers. Capsaicin reduces a body chemical that's important for sending pain messages.
- **Salicylates.** Salicylates (Bengay, Aspercreme, others) contain the pain-relieving substance found in aspirin.
- **Counterirritants.** Counterirritants (Biofreeze, Heet, others) contain substances such as menthol and camphor. These active ingredients produce a sensation of heat or cold that may temporarily override your ability to feel pain.

MOVEMENT AND EXERCISE

When your back or neck hurts, your instinct may be to move less. Instead of mowing the lawn or going shopping, you head for the couch or your favorite chair. But one of the best things you can do is to stay active. Physical activity gets blood flowing to your sore spots, loosening tight muscles and re-

leasing tension. It can also lift your mood and get your mind off your pain.

Daily activity

Try to keep up with your normal activities as much as possible. If you have a regular exercise routine, such as yoga, swimming or walking, stick with it as much as you can. If you don't exercise regularly, make an effort to keep your body moving.

If your pain is more severe, you may need to take it easy for a day or two by cutting back on certain activities or exercises. But try not to restrict your range of motion or stop moving completely out of fear of pain. Even if your pain is telling you to lie down, bed rest generally isn't recommended. Research shows that people who rest in bed take longer to recover than those who maintain their regular activities as much as possible.

Basic stretches

If you're feeling up for it, you might try doing some basic neck and back stretches. See Chapter 7 for stretches that you can do at home. Stretching helps improve flexibility and decrease tightness in the muscles that impact the neck and lower back.

By keeping your muscles limber, stretching can help relieve neck or back pain. It can also improve your overall range of motion and reduce the chances that you'll re-injure yourself in the future or develop a new injury.

LISTEN TO YOUR BODY

Let your body be your guide as you decide how much activity to include in your day. Some stiffness and soreness is to be expected, but don't push through activities, exercises, or stretches that cause an obvious spike in pain or worsen your condition.

Avoid painful movements, and if you need to, ease up on the intensity of your exercise routine. As the pain starts to improve, gradually return to your normal level of activity.

Before performing the stretches, you might try applying heat to the sore area to loosen tight muscles. If you have a sore neck, another option is to stand under a warm shower while you stretch.

Do the stretches slowly and gently without bouncing. The exercises shouldn't cause pain. If they do, stop and check that you're doing them correctly. Try the stretch again, but do it slowly and with less intensity. If the stretch is still painful, stop and talk to your doctor or a physical therapist before doing it again. For more information on physical therapy, see Chapter 7.

MASSAGE

If you've had a professional massage, you know how good it can feel. But you may be wondering whether a massage is helpful for back and neck conditions or if it could make the problems worse.

Massage is generally safe for people whose back or neck is hurting. It helps relieve pain and discomfort by reducing muscle tension and relieving stress. Research suggests that massage may improve short-term back and neck pain but is more useful for pain that's been lingering for four weeks or longer.

Massage basics

Massage is a general term for pressing, rubbing and manipulating your skin, muscles, tendons and ligaments. Massage may range from light stroking to deep pressure. No single type of massage is considered best for back and neck pain, so go with your personal preference. Common types of massage include:

- **Swedish massage.** This gentle form uses long strokes, kneading, deep circular movements, vibration and tapping to help relax and energize you.
- **Deep massage.** This massage technique uses slower, more-forceful strokes to target the deeper layers of muscle and connective tissue, commonly to help with muscle damage from injuries.
- **Sports massage.** It is similar to Swedish massage but is geared toward people involved in sports activities to help prevent or treat injuries.
- **Trigger point massage.** It focuses on areas of tight muscle fibers that can form in your muscles after injuries or overuse.

When seeking a massage therapist, ask your doctor or someone who you trust for a recommendation. Look for a therapist who's a licensed, reputable and experienced professional.

What to expect

Before your session starts, your massage therapist should ask you about any symptoms you're experiencing, your medical history and what you're hoping to get out of the massage. The therapist should explain the kind of massage and techniques he or she will use.

In a typical massage therapy session, you lie on a table and cover yourself with a sheet. You can also have a massage while sitting in a chair, fully clothed. Your massage therapist should perform an evaluation through touch to locate painful or tense areas and to determine how much pressure to apply.

Depending on your preference, your massage therapist may use oil or lotion to reduce friction on your skin. Let the therapist know if you're allergic to any ingredients.

A massage session may last from 15 to 90 minutes, depending on the type of massage performed and your available time. No matter what kind you choose, you should feel calm and relaxed during and after your massage. You shouldn't feel significant pain. If your therapist is pushing too hard on a sore spot, request lighter pressure.

After your massage, you may notice that your pain is improved and you're able to go about your daily activities more easily. However, these benefits tend to diminish over time. For that reason, some people find it helpful to receive regular massages while they're recovering.

COMMON QUESTIONS

You might have all sorts of questions about how to feel better and stay healthy. And there may be no lack of people offering you advice on what to try. Here are answers to questions that doctors commonly hear.

Should I wear a back brace?

If your back hurts, you might be wondering whether a back brace could give you added support while you heal. Perhaps you know people who swear by back braces, but you may have also heard reports that braces do more harm than good.

While some people find a brace helpful, scientific studies haven't been able to clearly show that braces effectively treat or prevent lower back pain. If overused, a back brace may even weaken the muscles that support your spine because the brace prevents the muscles from being used as much as they normally would. This can ultimately worsen back pain.

If you're considering wearing a back brace, talk to your medical provider. Back braces are available over-the-counter or by prescription. The most common types of braces include:

- **Corsets.** These back supports are similar in appearance to a traditional woman's corset. They're typically made of a soft, stretchy material such as cotton, nylon or neoprene and contain metal or plastic stays. They provide mild restriction of movement and may help to stabilize the back.
- **Back belts.** Like corsets, back belts are constructed with soft, stretchy materials, but they tend to be less flexible and are more restrictive to movement.
- **Semi-rigid and rigid braces (orthoses).** Orthoses are made with a combination of soft material and plastic or metal. They provide greater support than other back braces and significantly reduce range of motion. Rigid braces are often custom-made to fit a person's body.

Should I wear a neck brace?

If you're dealing with neck pain, wearing a neck brace for extra support might sound logical. However, research hasn't conclusively shown that neck braces (cervical collars) are an effective treatment for neck pain.

In some cases, neck braces may provide some relief during short bouts of increased pain, particularly at night when pain can disrupt your sleep. But they can also cause neck muscles to weaken from reduced use, prolonging your pain. Before wearing a neck brace, talk to your doctor and limit your use to no more than three hours a day for up to two weeks.

Will medical marijuana help relieve my pain?

As medical marijuana becomes more prevalent, this question is asked more often. Some research suggests that medical marijuana may be effective for treating chronic pain, especially pain caused by nerve damage. However, medical marijuana isn't recommended for back or neck pain because there aren't any high-quality studies showing that it's an effective treatment.

Keep in mind that possession of marijuana is illegal under federal law in the United States, but a majority of states have laws legalizing some form of medical marijuana, also called medical cannabis. The conditions that qualify for treatment with medical cannabis differ considerably among the states where it's legal. Some states have only a few qualifying conditions, while others have dozens.

If you're considering medical cannabis as a potential treatment for ongoing back or neck pain, talk with your medical provider. If your provider isn't familiar with medical cannabis, ask if there's another clinician in his or her practice who can answer your questions and help you understand potential benefits and risks.

Could my mattress be contributing to my back pain?

The jury is still out on this question. Several small studies focusing on chronic back pain suggest that medium-firm mattresses may be better for your back than firm mattresses. Adjustable air mattresses and mattresses topped with an inflatable overlay also may help reduce chronic back pain. Currently, no studies have focused on the link between mattress type and acute back pain. Experts agree that higher-quality research is needed to determine whether a specific level of firmness or mattress construction is best for preventing or improving back and neck conditions.

Is it true that sitting on my wallet can cause back problems?

Yes, it's true. Sitting on a wallet all day could be adding to your back woes. That's in part because sitting that way places your body in a lopsided position, with one hip higher than the other. This can throw your spine out of alignment. It may also put extra pressure on the pads (disks) between your vertebrae and on your sciatic nerve, the nerve that begins in your lower back and branches off down your hips, buttocks and each leg.

Sometimes, people who sit on their wallets for several hours start to notice a tingling or pain that radiates from the buttocks and down a leg. This condition even has a name: wallet sciatica, sometimes called wallet neuritis or fat wallet syndrome. The condition develops when a wallet compresses the sciatic nerve in the buttocks.

To protect your back, consider removing your wallet from your back pocket before sitting. Or keep it out of your back pocket altogether. If you think you may be experiencing the symptoms of wallet sciatica, talk to your doctor. Removing your wallet when you're sitting may relieve your discomfort.

Are heavy backpacks harmful?

If you or a child in your family lugs a backpack around, you may be wondering how heavy is too heavy. Most experts recommend that a backpack weigh no more than 10% of a person's body weight. With that said, studies on backpack use among school-aged children and teens don't definitively show that carrying a heavy backpack causes back or neck problems. But the quality of these studies is generally poor, and more research is needed.

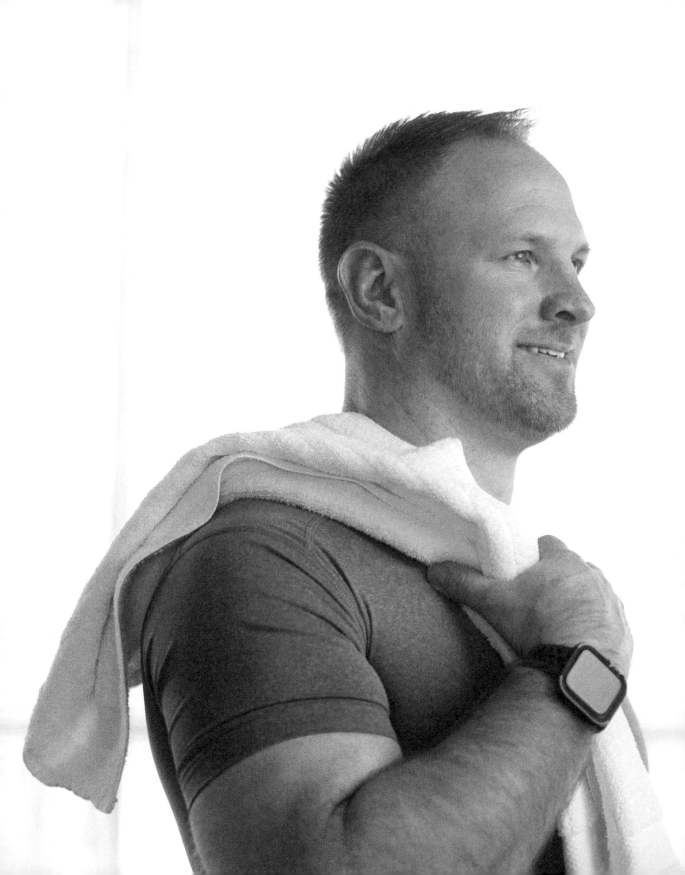

CHAPTER 7

Physical therapy

When your life is upended by a bout of back or neck pain, your initial reaction may be to lay low. Your goal is to move as little as possible because moving hurts. Despite your good intentions, this is the wrong approach. As you read in the previous chapter, to help your back or neck heal, you need to keep active.

While it may seem best to stay in bed or lie on the couch and wait for the pain to resolve, this has been shown to be counterproductive to the natural healing process.

In addition to helping reduce your pain, daily activity can help maintain or restore your flexibility, strength and endurance. In other words, instead of making your condition worse, movement can help improve it — provided you don't overdo it.

That said, you likely have a lot of questions. How much should you move? What exercises should you do? Are there things you should avoid? Is a little pain OK? What if it hurts a lot? This is where a physical therapist comes in. Many people who visit a doctor for back or neck pain are referred to physical therapy.

Physical therapy serves two main purposes — treatment and education. Physical therapists specialize in treating spinal conditions and other musculoskeletal problems. A physical therapist can instruct you on specific activities intended to help relieve subacute and chronic pain and build your strength. Physical therapists also provide education on daily exercises and other healthy lifestyle approaches to prevent future musculoskeletal problems.

Can you get better on your own without seeing a physical therapist? Yes. Often, the problem resolves on its own. But if your pain persists, a physical therapist will work with you to help relieve the pain and get you back to your normal activities. A therapist can also instruct you on steps you can take to help prevent a future recurrence.

SEEING A PHYSICAL THERAPIST

When your back or neck hurts and you see a doctor, he or she will try to determine what's triggering the pain. Sometimes the cause is evident, perhaps a pulled muscle or a ruptured (herniated) disk. Other times, it's not.

If your doctor isn't able to link your pain to a specific cause, he or she may refer you to physical therapy for additional evaluation and to see if specific activities may help remedy the problem. Your doctor may also recommend physical therapy when he or she knows what the problem is — what's causing your pain — but surgery isn't an option and other treatments haven't been helpful.

Most physical therapy sessions begin with an initial evaluation, in which the therapist is trying to get a detailed picture of your current condition and your overall health.

Pain history

At your first appointment, your physical therapist will likely want to gather informa-tion about your condition and your pain. Similar to your first appointment with your doctor, you may be asked to describe your symptoms, the location of your pain, the type of pain you have — shooting, burning, tingling, aching — and its severity. The therapist may ask if certain activities or positions worsen the pain or make it better.

Health history

Your therapist will want to get an idea of your overall health. This may include information about any medical conditions you may have and recent or past injuries. He or she also may inquire about your current level of activity. How active are you each day? Do you exercise regularly? What types of exercises do you do? Is it difficult for you to be active?

Physical exam

An examination typically follows. Your physical therapist may have you walk or perform certain movements, such as flexing forward or extending your upper body backward. He or she is paying attention to your spine and the structures that support it — muscles, tendons and ligaments. With the various tasks you're asked to do, your therapist is:

- Analyzing your body movements
- Testing your joints to see if they move the way they should
- Determining your flexibility
- Measuring your muscle strength

On occasion, a physical therapist may have you perform specific tests that require use of specialized equipment. Most often, though, a therapist can gather the information he or she needs just by having you move in certain ways.

It's important to keep in mind that just because you hurt doesn't mean that something is terribly wrong. Back and neck pain can be intense and persistent, but that doesn't necessarily indicate that you have a serious injury. In fact, it's not uncommon for a physical therapist or a doctor to find nothing wrong after a complete evaluation.

When the cause of your pain isn't evident, the plan of action is often to have you perform specific exercises or activities to see what helps. By learning which exercises improve your pain, your therapist can get a better idea of what might be triggering your discomfort.

FORMULATING A THERAPY PLAN

Based on the results of your health history and physical evaluation, your therapist will develop a personalized treatment plan with these goals in mind:

- Improve any structural impairments to your spine and pelvis
- Relieve or lessen your pain
- Return you to your normal activities as quickly as possible
- Improve your strength and your capacity to move without pain
- Improve your posture

Immediate care

Your treatment plan will likely include specific exercises that you perform daily or periodically throughout the week. The exercises you're asked to do will depend on your particular condition and what your therapist believes may be causing your discomfort.

Some exercises are designed to reduce irritation or pressure on your spine or a nerve. Others are intended to improve flexibility and limber up overly tight muscles. A physical therapist may perform hands-on treatment, such as soft tissue and joint manipulation, to improve your flexibility and limber up your muscles.

In the past, physical therapy frequently included treatments such as ultrasound or electrical stimulation. These interventions are less commonly used today because studies haven't found strong evidence that they're helpful over the long term. For back and neck pain, a treatment plan that emphasizes activity and movement is generally the most beneficial.

If the deep (core) muscles that help support your spine are weak, you may be prescribed exercises to help strengthen those muscles. If your posture is a problem, your plan may include exercises to improve your posture.

Considerations

When formulating a personalized therapy plan, your physical therapist will take into account practical considerations, including facility and staff availability, your fitness level, personal preferences, and past history.

Topics discussed may include: Do you have access to a nearby gym, physical therapist or trainer? Can you perform the exercises on your own at home? Do you have someone to help you, if assistance is needed? Are you more likely to do the exercises if someone is there to supervise you? Some people prefer a more structured approach with assistance from an expert, while others would rather do the activities independently.

Future care

In addition to exercises to help relieve your pain, your physical therapist may devise a broader exercise program to improve your overall health and reduce the likelihood of your symptoms recurring. Keeping active with day-to-day activities such as walking, light exercise and household chores is helpful, and you want to keep doing them. But you may also benefit from more-structured exercise.

Studies suggest that regular aerobic activity is good for your back and neck. Researchers have found that people with chronic back pain who regularly participate in moderate to vigorous aerobic activities have less pain and function better compared with individuals who are less physically active.

Exercise also provides neurological and psychological benefits. It releases natural painkillers and feel-good hormones called endorphins and enkephalins. These chemicals give you an increased sense of well-being and help lessen feelings of stress, anxiety and depression. In addition to helping you move better, exercise helps you to feel better.

BACK EXERCISES

Your personal physical therapy plan may include one or more of the following:
• Stretching and flexibility exercises
• Core strengthening exercises

For each exercise that you're asked to do, a therapist will teach you how to do it correctly and instruct you on how often to perform the exercise. On pages 109-120 are examples of some exercises that your physical therapist may recommend.

Stretching (flexibility) exercises

Your ability to move normally and comfortably is dependent on the flexibility of several key muscle groups of the spine, hips and lower extremities. Stretching exercises are intended to keep those key muscles limber. (See the exercises on pages 109-115.)

Stretching exercises should be done gently, holding each stretch for about 30 to 60 seconds. Your therapist will instruct you on how often to do them and how many repetitions of each stretch you should do. Repetitions may increase gradually over time.

IT WON'T HURT YOU

People bothered by back and neck problems are often a bit leery of embarking on an exercise routine. They worry that exercise isn't safe and more activity will only make their problems worse. You may be especially concerned if you've been told that you have an "unstable" spine, "misaligned" vertebrae or a "bulging" disk. These terms can be frightening and may lead you to believe that one wrong move or misstep and you're in real trouble!

For most people, there is nothing to fear. Exercise won't worsen your condition. In fact, it should do the opposite. In some instances, depending on your situation and what could be triggering your pain, there may be specific movements or activities that your physical therapist suggests you avoid. For the most part, though, exercise won't harm you. That said, you need to be smart. For example, if your back hurts, try and avoid activities over the short-term that place excessive stress on your lower back, such as heavy lifting. When your pain improves, you should be able to gradually return to activities such as lifting, bending and prolonged sitting.

A physical therapist can answer your questions about what activities are safe for you to do and which you might want to avoid. When starting an activity program, you may have a bit more discomfort. Muscles, tendons, ligaments and other structures that you haven't been using need to get used to being active again. But you shouldn't experience severe or sharp pain. If you do, stop what you're doing.

Also remember that you should avoid any stretch that is too difficult for you to do or that causes pain when you perform it. Stretching may produce some tension or feel a bit uncomfortable, especially when you first get started, but it shouldn't cause pain.

Core strengthening exercises

Core exercises are a key component of a well-rounded fitness program and are especially important to back and neck health. However, aside from occasional situps and pushups, core exercises are often neglected.

Your body's core muscles support and help protect your spine. These muscle groups include the hip, pelvic, abdominal and back muscles. If your core muscles are weak, your spine isn't getting the support that it needs to keep it stable. A stronger core allows you to be more active without experiencing pain.

A physical therapist will work with you on specific exercises to help strengthen your core muscles. Core exercises train the muscles in your pelvis, lower back, hips and abdomen to work in harmony. This leads to better balance and stability, whether doing routine activities or spending time on the basketball or tennis court. In fact, most sports and physical activities depend on stable core muscles.

Strong core muscles make it easier to perform many tasks, such as swing a golf club, get a glass from the top shelf and bend down to tie your shoes. Strong core muscles are also important for athletes, such as runners, as weak core muscles can increase fatigue, reduce endurance and produce more injuries.

A physical therapist will instruct you on proper technique to safely start and progress with these exercises, including how many of the exercises you should do in one sitting. It's best to start slowly and gradually progress to include additional exercises or more repetitions.

Similar to stretching exercises, make sure to avoid any core strengthening exercises that you find too difficult or that cause pain when you perform them.

On pages 116-120 are some examples of core strengthening exercises your therapist may recommend.

NECK EXERCISES

Physical therapy is also fundamental to the treatment of many neck conditions. A physical therapist can teach you correct posture, alignment and neck strengthening exercises to help ease your neck pain or prevent a recurrence.

Similar to exercises recommended to help treat back pain, the exercises that your therapist recommends to ease your neck pain will depend on your condition and health history. For each exercise that you're asked to do, your therapist will teach you how to do it correctly and instruct you on how often to do it.

On pages 121-125 are examples of some basic neck exercises that your physical therapist may recommend.

If you're bothered by neck pain, it's also important that you maintain your core strength. If your core muscles aren't strong, your neck and shoulder muscles may be overworked.

In addition, for neck pain as well as back pain, practicing good posture is important and can help relieve your pain.

LOWER BACK GLUTEAL STRETCH

1. Lie on your back on a firm, flat surface.
2. Put your hands below one knee and gently pull your knee to your chest until you feel a stretch in your lower back. Don't bounce.
3. Hold the stretch and then slowly return to the starting position.
4. Repeat the stretch with the other leg.

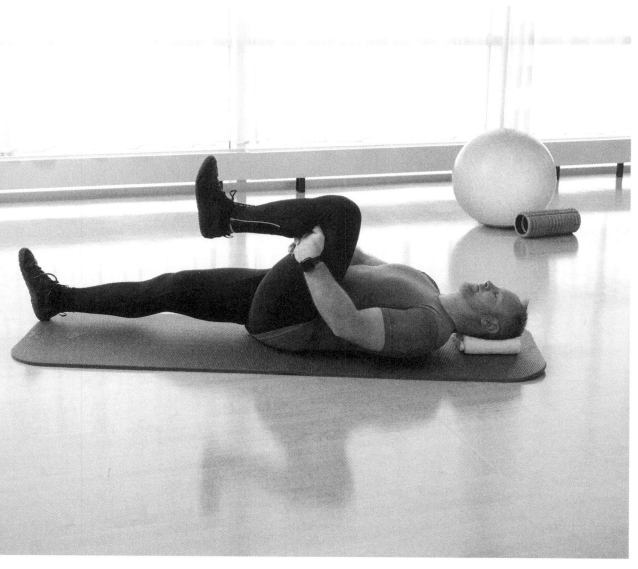

LUMBAR STRETCH

1. Lie on your back on a firm, flat surface.
2. Lifting one leg at a time, put your hands below your knees and gently pull both knees to your chest until you feel a stretch in your lower back. Don't bounce.
3. Hold the stretch and then slowly return to the starting position.

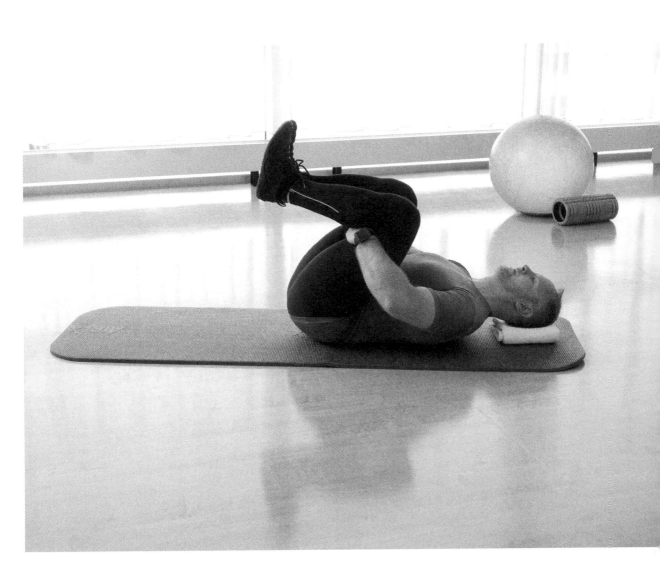

PIRIFORMIS STRETCH

1. Sitting on the edge of a bench or chair, place one foot on the knee of the opposite leg.
2. Lean forward and bring your upper body down toward your knee until you feel a stretch in your buttock. Don't bounce.
3. Hold the stretch and then slowly return to the starting position.
4. Repeat the stretch using your other leg.

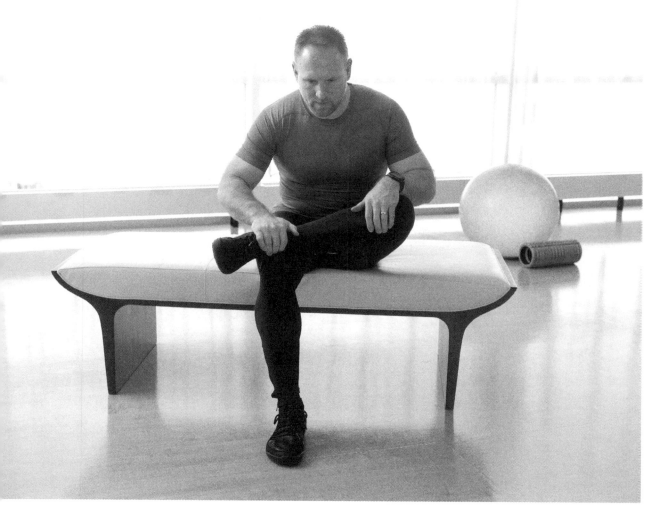

CAT STRETCH

1. Kneel on your knees and hands on a firm, flat surface.
2. Slowly arch your back away from the surface as you bring your head down. Hold the stretch.
3. Slowly let you back sag toward the surface as you bring your head back and chin up. Hold the stretch.
4. Return to the starting position.

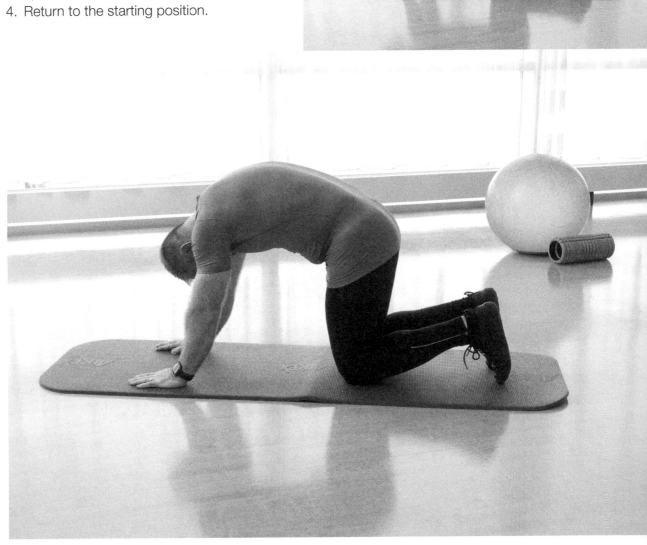

LUMBAR ROTATION STRETCH

1. Lie on your back on a firm, flat surface. Bend your legs at the knee so that your feet are flat on the surface.
2. Keeping your head and shoulders on the surface, slowly roll your knees and hips to one side until you feel a stretch in your lower back. Don't bounce.
3. Hold the stretch and then slowly return to the starting position.
4. Do this stretch on the other side.

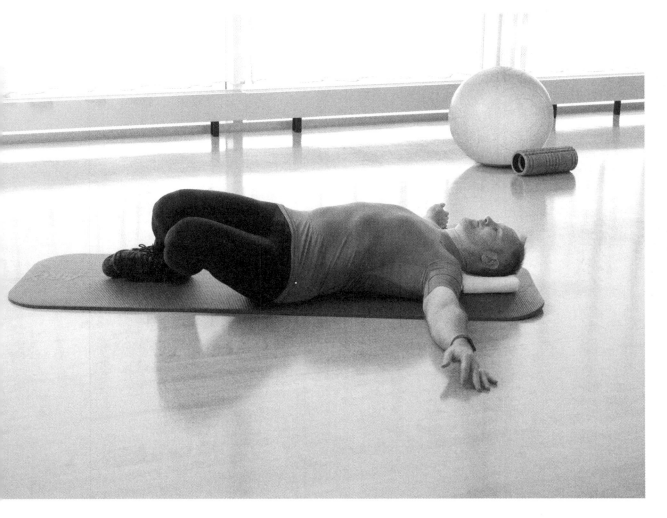

KNEELING LUMBAR STRETCH

1. Kneel on your hands and knees on a firm, flat surface.
2. Bring your chin down and slowly sit back on your heels as you bring your arms out in front of you until you feel a stretch in your lower back. Don't bounce.
3. Hold the stretch and then slowly return to the starting position.

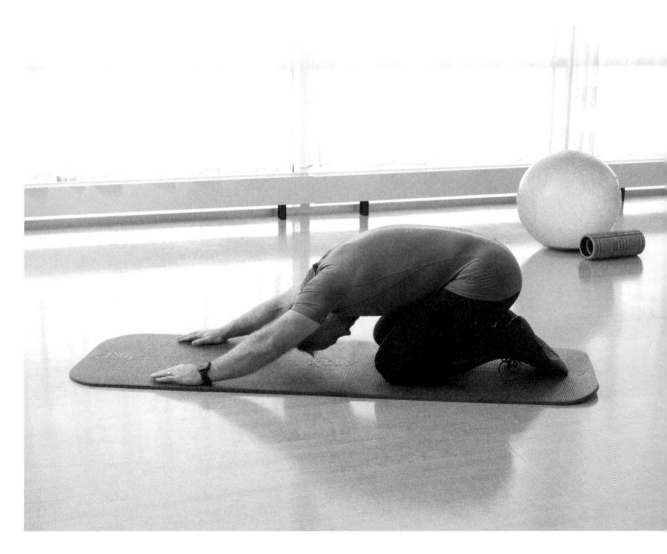

SITTING LUMBAR STRETCH

1. Sit on a chair.
2. Bring your chin toward your chest, and slowly bend forward as you bring your hands toward the floor until you feel a stretch in your lower back. Keep your elbows between your knees and don't bounce.
3. Hold the stretch and then slowly return to the starting position.

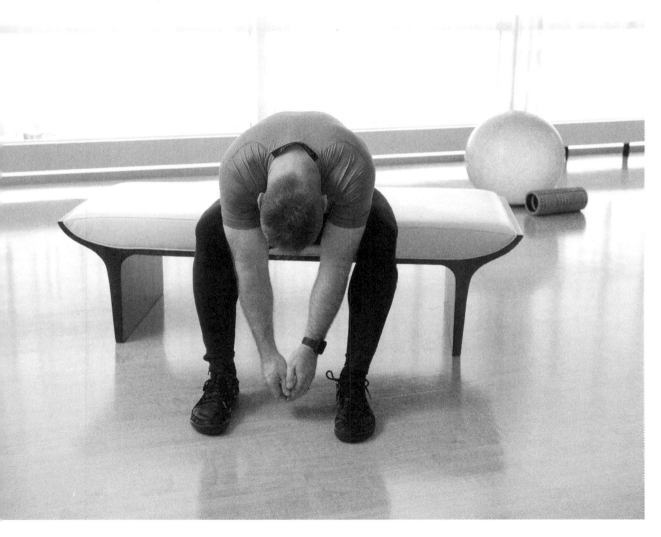

STABILIZATION PLANK

1. Lie on your stomach propped up on your forearms with your chin tucked in and your feet together.
2. While maintaining this position, tighten your abdominal muscles.
3. Hold the position briefly, relax and repeat.

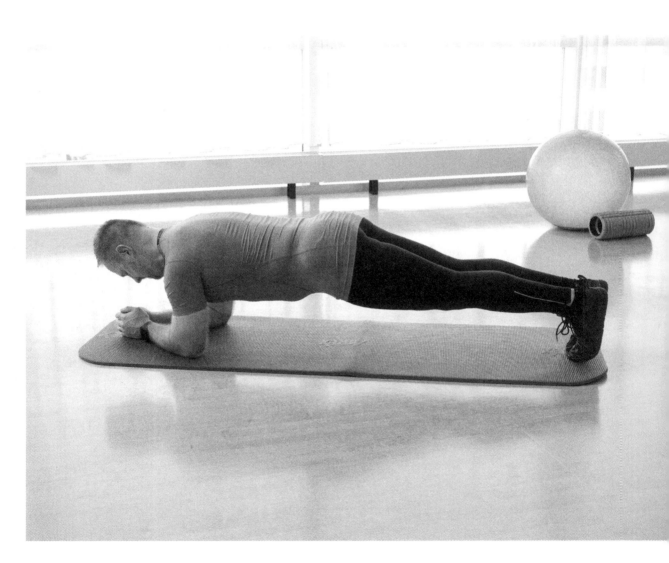

ABDOMINAL BRACING

1. Lie on your back on a firm, flat surface with your knees bent, your feet flat on the surface and your back in neutral (slightly arched) position.
2. Place your hands on your lower abdomen and breathe steadily through your abdomen. Tighten your abdominal muscles so that your navel moves inward toward your spine. At the same time, engage your pelvic floor muscles. Flex the muscles the same as you would to stop urinating or stop passing gas.
3. You should feel slow, deep tension under your fingers. Your rib cage should not become rigid and your pelvis should not move.
4. Hold the position briefly, relax and repeat several times.

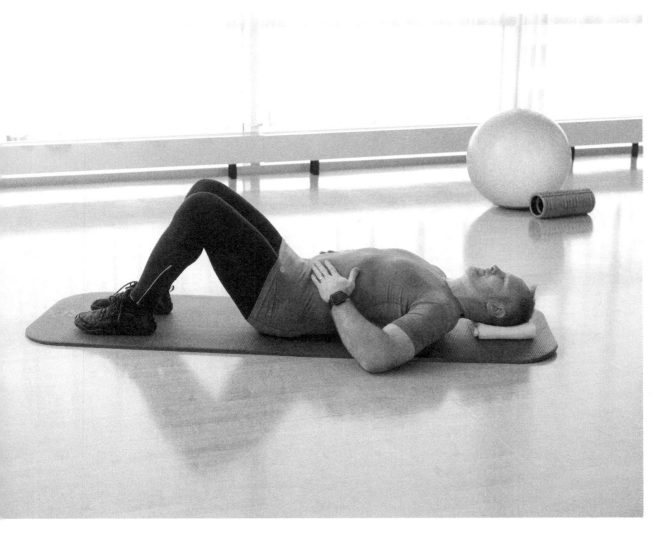

BIRD DOG

1. Get on your hands and knees with your knees directly under your hips and your hands directly under your shoulders.
2. Your back should be in a neutral (slightly arched) position and your chin tucked in.
3. Slightly tighten your abdominal muscles and lumbar muscles and extend one leg behind you while keeping your back and pelvis still.
4. Extend the opposite arm in front while keeping your balance.
5. Try to grab something in front of you with your hand and touch an imaginary wall behind the foot of your extended leg.
6. Hold the position and then slowly return to the starting position.
7. Repeat with the other leg and arm.
8. Begin with a few repetitions and slowly add repetitions as the exercise becomes easier.

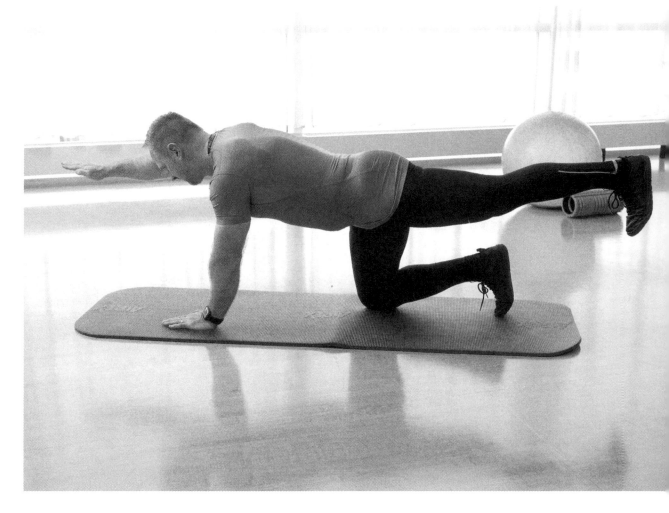

BRIDGE

1. Lie on your back on a firm, flat surface with your knees bent and feet flat on the surface. Tighten your abdominal muscles and keep them tight during the exercise.
2. Squeeze your buttocks together and lift them off the ground to make a straight line with your body. Only your head, should-ers, and feet or heels should be touching the surface.
3. You should feel tension in your buttocks, thighs and abdomen.
4. Hold the position briefly and return to the starting position.

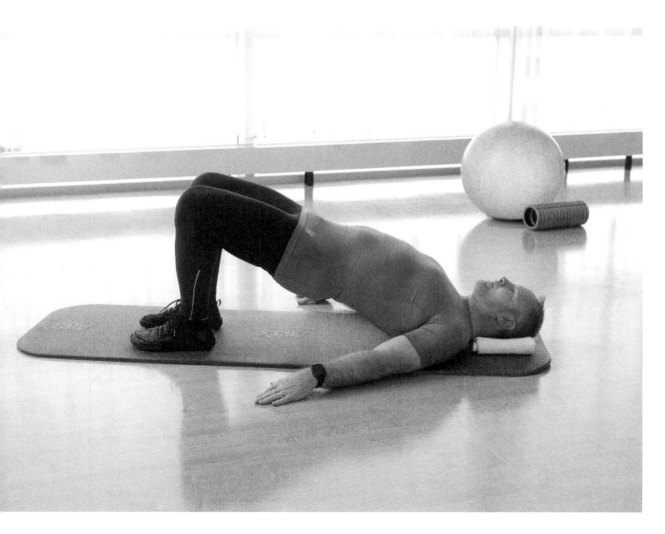

STABILIZATION SQUAT

1. Stand with both feet hip-width apart in front of a chair or bench.
2. While keeping your back straight and your kneecaps pointed straight ahead, slowly lower your body into a seated position (90-degree angle) on the chair or bench. Your heels should remain flat on the ground.
3. Push your weight into your heels and use your gluteal muscles to return to your initial, standing position.
4. Repeat until you feel fatigued in your thighs or buttocks, or both.

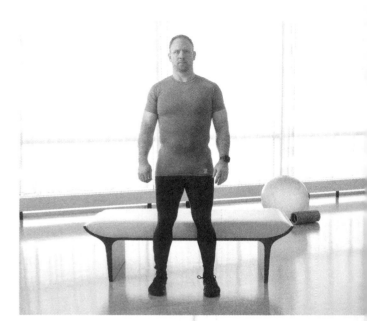

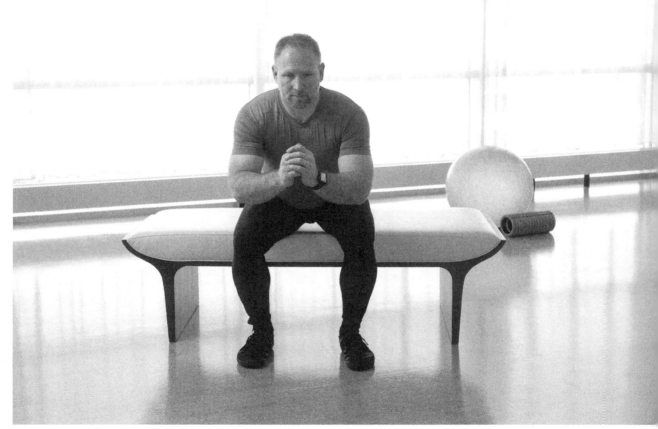

CHIN TUCK

1. Face forward, keeping your chin tucked in.
2. Nod your head around an imaginary axis through yours ears, slowly gliding your head backward and upward.
3. Hold several seconds and repeat.
4. This can easily be incorporated into daily activities, especially when you're seated.

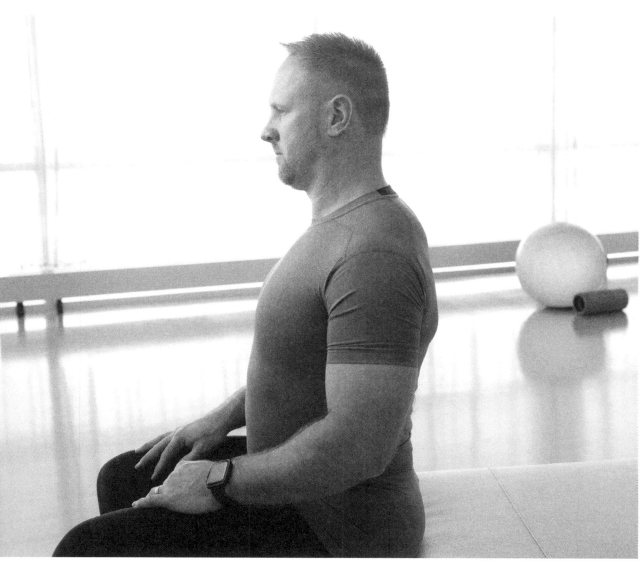

PECTORAL STRETCH LYING DOWN

1. Lie on your back on a firm, flat surface. Bend your knees so that your feet are flat on the surface.
2. Spread your arms out.
3. Bend your arms at your elbows and rest your arms on the flat surface.
4. Hold briefly and return to the starting position.
5. Bend your arms at your elbows and place your hands under your head.
6. Gently push your elbows toward the flat surface.
7. Hold the position briefly and return to the starting position.

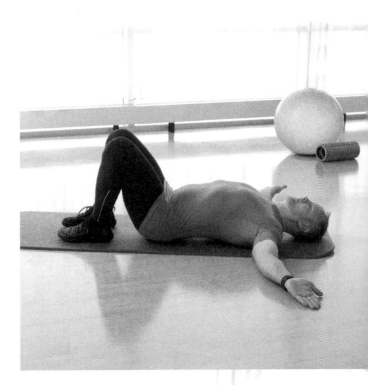

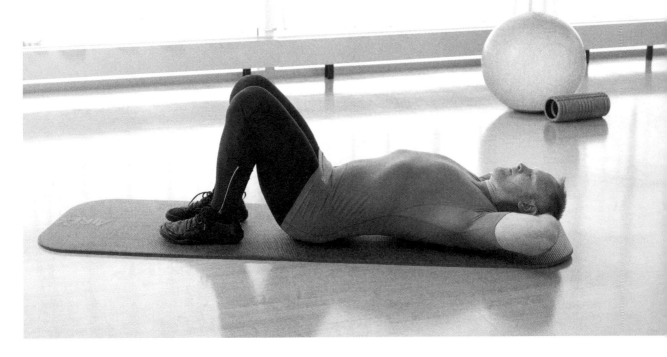

SHOULDER BLADES SQUEEZE

1. Sit or stand straight facing forward.
2. Pull your shoulder blades down and together behind you.
3. Hold the squeeze briefly and return to the starting position.

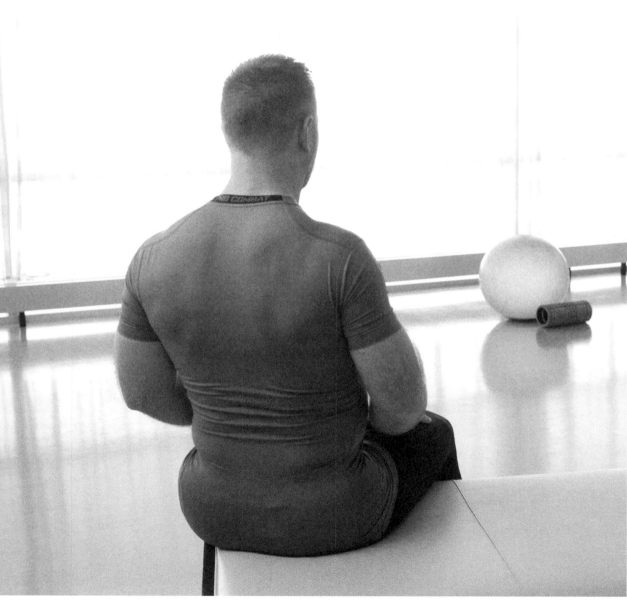

STANDING PECTORAL STRETCH

1. Stand in a comfortable stance inside a doorway. A corner where two walls meet also will work (as pictured).
2. Place one of your hands on the door frame or wall, keeping your elbow lower than your shoulder.
3. As you move one leg forward, slowly push your upper body forward to feel a stretch in your shoulders and chest. Keep your head in line with your body.
4. Hold briefly and return to the starting position.

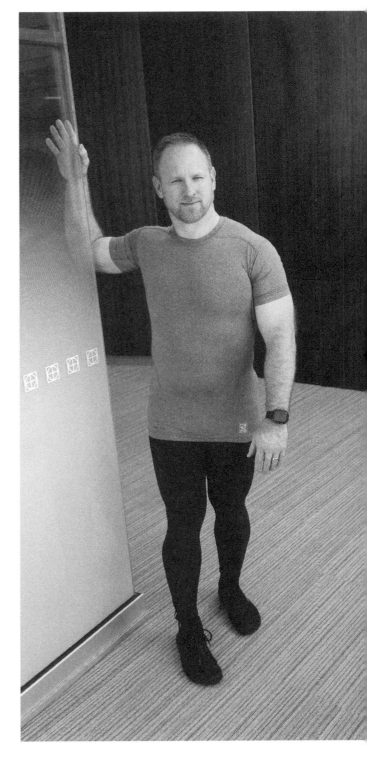

TRAPEZIUS STRETCH

1. Bend your head to your right.
2. Place your right hand on top and around your head for support. Don't pull on your head with the right hand.
3. Place your left hand adjacent to your left hip, grasping a chair or bench.
4. Slowly lean forward and to the right, pulling your left shoulder down. You'll feel a stretch along the left side of your neck.
5. Hold the stretch and slowly return to the starting position.
6. Change your position and do the stretch on the other side.

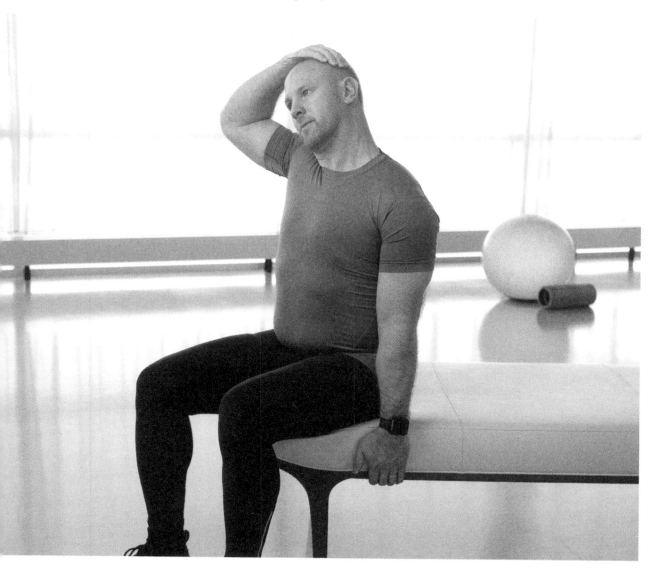

HOW MANY SESSIONS?

How often you need to see a physical therapist can vary widely. For some people, one visit may be enough. Others may need to see a physical therapist regularly over a period of a few weeks or months.

The optimal number of physical therapy sessions often is dependent on your condition and its severity, and how good you are at exercising on your own. Some people prefer to do their stretching and strengthening exercises at home or at a gym, and they're compliant in doing them each day. Others would rather have the support and guidance of a physical therapist. Or they know that if left to their own, chances are good they'll find excuses and not do the exercises.

If you do see a physical therapist regularly, check to see how many sessions your health insurance will cover.

POSTURE AND ERGONOMICS

Treating back and neck pain goes beyond exercises. Your physical therapist may spend time teaching you good habits and principles related to posture and ergonomics.

Posture

Good posture places only minimal strain on your joints and muscles. Poor posture, on the other hand, can increase stress on some muscles, stretching them or causing them to shorten. When overstretched, your muscles lose their strength and are more prone to injury and pain.

Learning and practicing proper posture can help relax your muscles and may reduce your pain. Throughout the day, including when you sit, stand and exercise, you want to maintain good posture. A physical therapist can give you tips on how to do that.

Don't be surprised if your therapist also asks about your sleeping positions and the pillows you use. Your back and neck need proper support during sleep, just like they do while you're sitting or standing. While sleeping, you want to try and keep your spine aligned and your neck and back supported. That's why a visit to a physical therapist may include a discussion of good sleep positions, proper head and neck support,

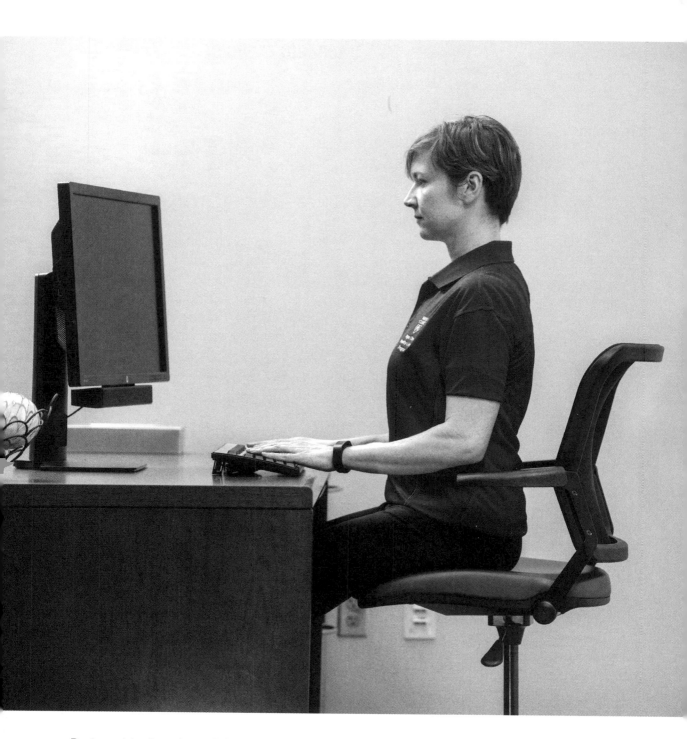

Posture. Ideally, when sitting, your back should be straight, your shoulders should be pulled back, and your elbows bent with your arms at your sides and your wrists neutral.

and use of pillows to help keep your neck and back in alignment.

Ergonomics

Ergonomics basically involves making sure that your workspace allows you to do your job safely and efficiently. A physical therapist may ask you what you do most of the day — sit, stand, lift, walk and so on — to determine if you have proper support and if you are using safe techniques when doing these tasks.

For example, if you sit behind a desk for hours at a time, you don't want to be doomed to a career of neck and back pain or sore wrists and fingers. Proper office ergonomics — including correct chair height, proper placement of equipment such as a computer and keyboard, and good desk posture — can help you and your joints stay comfortable at work.

For people who sit a lot, it's also important to get up every so often and move, stretch or walk. Prolonged sitting can lead to weakened muscles and increase your risk of back and neck problems. The same is true if your job requires that you stand in one location for lengthy periods or perform repetitive tasks. Frequent breaks can help reduce your risk of injury.

For more information on proper posture, including information and illustrations on how to sit, stand and lift properly, see Chapter 10.

AEROBIC EXERCISE

Aerobic exercise is good for your back and your neck. Studies show that regular aerobic activity can help reduce subacute and chronic back pain — pain lasting for more than four weeks. More importantly, aerobic exercise can help prevent future back and neck problems.

Aerobic exercises are those that are low enough in intensity that they can be maintained for long periods — 30 to 60 minutes — but high enough in intensity that your heart rate and breathing increase while you do them, and you may sweat. Examples of aerobic exercise include brisk walking, jogging, riding a bicycle, swimming and dancing.

If you're not physically active, beyond stretching and strengthening exercises, your physical therapist may recommend a program of aerobic activity to help manage your condition and prevent future recurrences.

Some people have problems getting started with aerobic activities or sticking with them. Think about your exercise obstacles — lack of interest, inaccessibility to a gym, cost, too little time, self-consciousness, embarrassment, anxiety or frustration. Now do some strategizing. What would make exercise more enjoyable to you, so that you'd do it? It might be the type of activity. Do what you enjoy. Maybe you're not into jogging or bicycling, but you like pickleball or water aerobics. Perhaps you need an exercise buddy, someone to keep you motivated and accountable.

For many people, the simplest way to include more aerobic activity in their day is to walk. If you haven't exercised a lot and following an exercise routine is new to you, walking might be a good way to start. You can read about how to begin a walking program, along with other exercise options, in Chapter 10.

The decision to become more active is an investment in yourself, your family and your future — and the rewards are enormous. Far beyond simply managing back and neck pain, regular aerobic exercise can help you control your weight, improve your coordination and balance, reduce muscle aches and pains, avoid insomnia, and prevent or delay many diseases and conditions, including diabetes, heart disease and cancer.

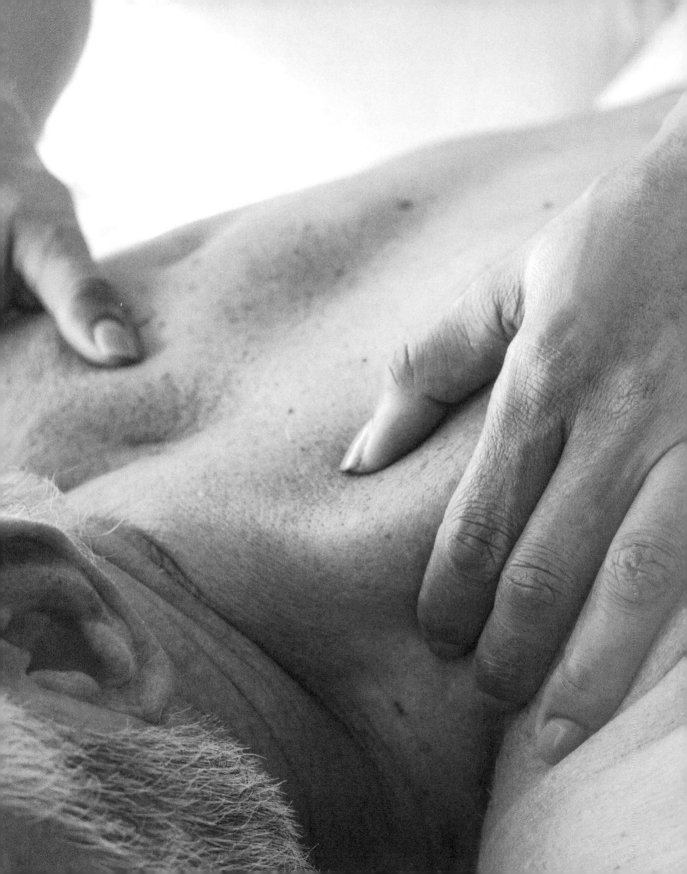

CHAPTER 8

Nonsurgical interventions

If you've been dealing with a back or neck condition that's not getting better, you might be starting to lose hope. It's hard to keep your chin up when pain seems to creep into every corner of your life. You desperately want to feel normal again and wonder if that will ever happen.

As you learned in Chapters 6 and 7, exercise and physical therapy can go a long way toward helping many people recover from their back and neck problems, and these treatments are often a good place to start. But sometimes they aren't enough to fully relieve your pain and heal your body.

Fortunately, there are many other nonsurgical interventions that can jump-start a stalled recovery and help you feel better. Nonsurgical treatments include chiropractic care and acupuncture to injections, nerve stimulation and medication — and there are more treatment options on the horizon.

This chapter will walk you through a variety of nonsurgical interventions for back and neck problems. You'll learn when these treatments are commonly used, how they can help and whether there are potential downsides. With guidance from your doctor, you may be able to take advantage of one or more of these treatments so that you can get a handle on your pain and get your life back on track.

CHIROPRACTIC CARE

When back or neck pain strikes, some people quickly turn to a chiropractor in hopes of finding relief. Others are more cautious.

They've heard that chiropractic care may be helpful, but don't know much about it or what to expect.

The goal of chiropractic care is to restore spinal movement and, as a result, reduce back or neck pain and improve daily functioning. During a chiropractic adjustment, also known as spinal manipulation, trained specialists use their hands or a small instrument to apply a controlled, sudden force to a spinal joint. They may also use muscle pressure and stretching to relax muscles that are tightened or in spasm.

Chiropractic care is based on the idea that your body's structure — nerves, bones, joints and muscles — and its capacity for healthy function are closely intertwined. By aligning and balancing your body's structure, chiropractic treatment is intended to support the body's natural ability to heal itself. Chiropractic care is most commonly practiced by chiropractors, but doctors of osteopathic medicine and some physical therapists also perform this treatment.

When chiropractic care is an option

Chiropractic care may be worth considering if you have mild to moderate back and neck pain caused by muscle strain, inflammation or muscle spasms. This type of treatment

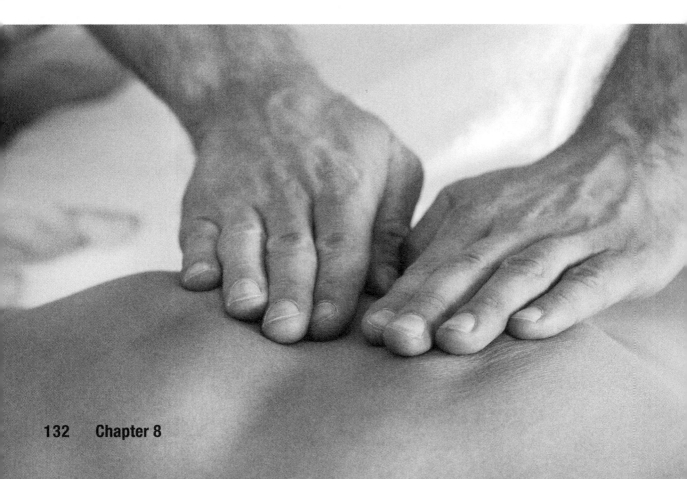

may also help relieve pain caused by compression of the sciatic nerve (sciatica), especially when used in conjunction with physical therapy and exercise. But chiropractic care isn't appropriate for everyone. Chiropractic adjustment isn't advised if you have:

- Severe osteoporosis
- Loss of strength in an arm or leg
- Cancer in your spine
- An increased risk of stroke
- Narrowed and hardened arteries (atherosclerosis) in the neck
- Inflammatory arthritis

If you're uncertain whether chiropractic care is right for you, talk to your doctor. He or she may also be able to recommend a good chiropractor or other specialist.

Effectiveness and safety

Studies examining the effectiveness of chiropractic care show that it can reduce or relieve pain in some people with back or neck conditions. Chiropractic treatment may be most effective when used with other treatments, such as physical therapy or regular exercise.

Chiropractic adjustments are generally considered safe for back and neck conditions when they're performed by someone who's trained and licensed to deliver chiropractic care. You may have mild soreness or aching following treatment, just as you would with some forms of exercise. But this soreness usually resolves within 12 to 48 hours after treatment.

Serious complications associated with chiropractic adjustment are rare. They may include a herniated disk or worsening of an existing disk herniation, or a compression of the nerves in your lower spinal column (cauda equina syndrome). In very rare instances, neck manipulation may cause a type of stroke known as vertebral artery dissection.

If you seek out chiropractic care, the number of treatment sessions you'll need will depend on the severity of your pain. If your pain doesn't improve after two to three sessions, or if it gets worse, talk to your doctor. You may be better off stopping chiropractic care in favor of other treatments.

ACUPUNCTURE

Acupuncture is another treatment you've likely heard of but may not know a lot about. Acupuncture involves the insertion of very thin needles to various depths at strategic points on your body. Some people with back and neck conditions find acupuncture helpful, especially when it's done in combination with other treatments.

During an acupuncture session, between five and 20 needles may be inserted while you sit or lie on a padded table. Most people feel only minimal pain or pressure as the needles are inserted; some feel nothing at all. Once the needles are in place, you generally shouldn't feel any pain. Your practitioner may gently move or twirl the needles after placement or apply heat or mild electrical pulses to the needles. There is usually no discomfort when the needles are removed.

How acupuncture works isn't entirely understood. Traditional Chinese medicine explains acupuncture as a technique for balancing the flow of energy or life force — known as chi or qi (chee) — that is believed to flow through pathways (meridians) in your body. By inserting needles at specific points along these meridians, acupuncture practitioners believe that your energy flow will re-balance.

In contrast, many Western practitioners view the acupuncture points as places to stimulate nerves, muscles and connective tissue. Some believe that this stimulation boosts your body's natural painkillers.

When acupuncture is an option

Because acupuncture has low risks and few side effects, it may be worth a try if you're dealing with persistent pain in your back or neck, including muscle (myofascial) pain. But acupuncture isn't suitable in certain situations. You may be at risk of complications if you:

- Have a bleeding disorder or are taking blood thinners
- Have a pacemaker
- Are pregnant

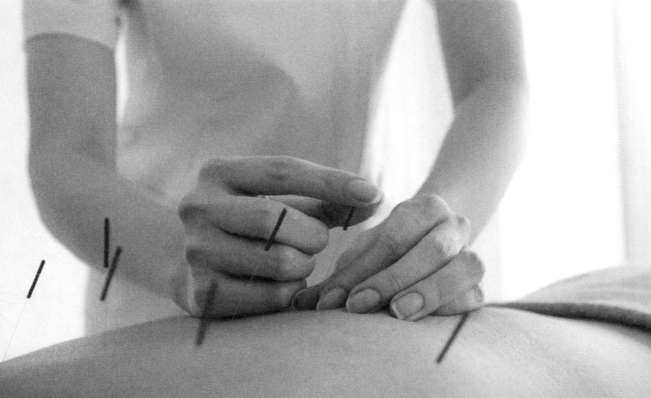

Effectiveness and safety

The benefits of acupuncture are sometimes difficult to measure, but studies suggest that acupuncture may reduce pain for some people with back and neck problems.

The risks of acupuncture are low if you're working with a competent, certified acupuncture practitioner. Common side effects include soreness or minor bleeding or bruising where the needles were inserted. Single-use, disposable needles are now the practice standard, so the risk of infection is small.

If you're considering acupuncture, don't be afraid to talk to your doctor. He or she may help you determine if acupuncture is a good option for you and recommend a practitioner. You can also ask other people you trust for recommendations.

It's important to work with a qualified practitioner. Check the practitioner's training and credentials. Most states require that acupuncturists who aren't physicians pass an exam conducted by the National Certification Commission for Acupuncture and Oriental Medicine.

The number of acupuncture sessions needed differs from person to person and depends on how severe your pain is. You should experience some pain relief within the first few weeks. If your symptoms don't start to improve, then it may be time to discuss other treatment options with your doctor.

INJECTIONS

If you've tried physical therapy and other conservative treatments but you're still dealing with debilitating and persistent pain, your doctor may recommend injection therapy at the source of your pain. Injections generally don't cure pain, but they may help you through an initial period of intense pain or a flare-up of severe pain. Pain relief from injection therapy may also help to speed your recovery if it allows you to participate more actively in physical therapy, exercise and other parts of your treatment program.

Your doctor may suggest injection therapy if your pain is associated with a spinal joint, nerve or muscle that's been damaged, is irritated, or is inflamed. Injections are typically given by a spine specialist or a pain medication specialist with expertise in therapeutic injections.

Receiving an injection

Most injections generally include an anesthetic and a steroid medication. During the procedure, you'll lie facedown on your stomach on the examining table. Your doctor may use fluoroscopy, an X-ray imaging procedure, that allows him or her to view the spinal column as the injection needle containing medication is inserted at the site of your pain. You may feel some discomfort or pain during the injections. If you feel a lot of pain, tell your doctor. The injection procedure itself usually takes about 15 minutes,

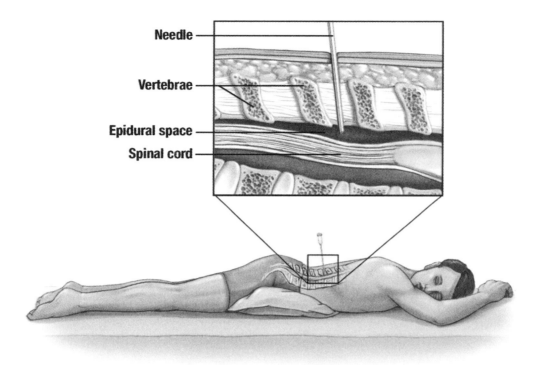

Needle

Vertebrae

Epidural space

Spinal cord

Epidural injection. An epidural injection is an injection of medication into the space around the spinal nerves, also known as the epidural space.

---

but your appointment will likely last longer than that, possibly several hours.

Anesthetic The anesthetic medication lidocaine is commonly used to temporarily numb a painful area. It works by interfering with, or blocking, pain pathways to the brain. The result is less pain in that area for a short period.

An anesthetic may be injected in combination with a steroid medication to lower the amount of pain you feel during the injection procedure and right after it. The anesthetic usually wears off within two to eight hours.

Sometimes doctors use anesthetic-only injections to help diagnose the cause of your pain. Suppose, for example, that a small amount of an anesthetic injected at a specific location relieves your pain. This indicates that a particular joint or nerve may be the source of the pain. If, on the other hand, the injection doesn't reduce your pain, you may receive another injection in a different location during another office visit.

Once your doctor has located the source of your pain, he or she may recommend a steroid injection at the source or suggest a different treatment option.

Steroid Long-acting injected steroid medications help decrease pain by reducing inflammation in joints or muscles and around nerves. In the short term, steroids can make you feel dramatically better and they may provide pain relief for two to four months.

However, when used for many months or years, there's a chance that steroid injections could cause serious side effects, including weakened joints and cartilage, diabetes, high blood pressure, osteoporosis, damaged adrenal glands, and decreased ability to heal wounds and fight infections. For this reason, your doctor may recommend no more than three or four steroid injections a year.

Injection locations

Injections for back and neck conditions may be given in a variety of locations along the spine. The site of your injection will depend on the cause and source of your pain. Below are some of the more common locations for back and neck conditions.

Epidural An epidural injection is the most common type of injection for back and neck pain. In this procedure, a needle containing medication is inserted into the epidural space that surrounds the spinal cord and spinal nerves. The medication coats nerves in the location where it's injected, relieving pain.

Your doctor may recommend an epidural if you have severe nerve pain that radiates down your arms, legs or buttocks as a result of conditions such as spinal stenosis or a damaged or bulging (herniated) disk.

Types of epidural injections include:
- **Interlaminar.** With this epidural technique, the needle is inserted between the bones of the spine to deliver medication near an inflamed or irritated nerve in the neck or back.
- **Transforaminal.** This approach involves inserting the needle through an opening at the side of the spine where a nerve root is exiting the vertebrae. The transforaminal technique is most commonly used to place medication close to an inflamed or irritated nerve root in the back, but in some cases your doctor may recommend it for neck pain.
- **Caudal.** This injection is guided into the caudal epidural space, located at the base of the spine below the lower end of the spinal cord. It may be used for low back pain that is caused by activities such as prolonged sitting or lifting heavy weights.

Facet joint Facet joints are small joints located in pairs at each vertebral level of the spine. The joints connect one vertebra to another, helping to stabilize your spine and allowing you to bend and twist.

Facet joints rub together when you move. As you age, the wear and tear from this movement can damage the joints, sometimes leading to facet joint disease. This condition can cause chronic pain in your neck, back or buttocks. Trauma or injury to the spine, such as from whiplash, is another cause of facet joint pain.

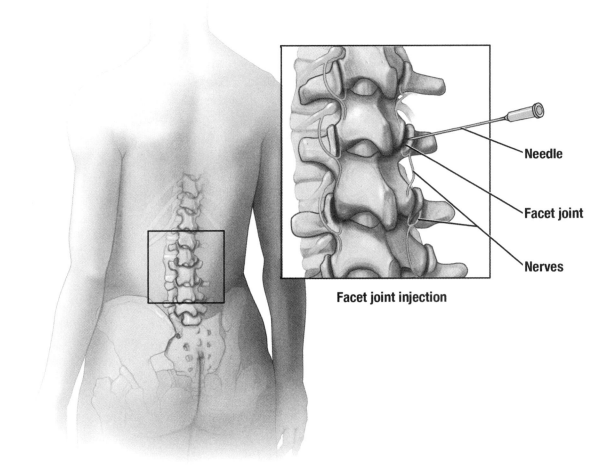

Needle

Facet joint

Nerves

Facet joint injection

Facet joint injection. Medications used in facet joint injections may be injected into the joint or into the medial branch nerves that supply the facet joints.

A facet joint injection delivers medication to or near a painful joint. It may relieve your pain by reducing inflammation and swelling in your joint.

Sacroiliac joint These injections are directed to a sacroiliac joint, a large joint located in your lower back and pelvic region. You have a sacroiliac joint on the right and left sides of your lower back that support the weight of your upper body when you stand.

Sacroiliac joint injections may help to treat low back or buttock pain caused by an in-

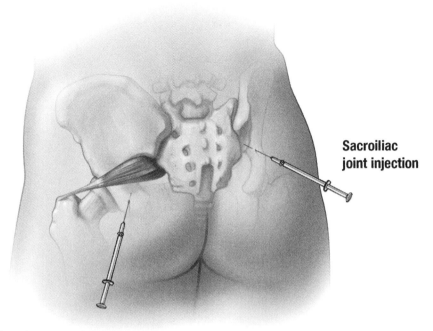

Sacroiliac joint injection

Piriformis muscle injection

Piriformis muscle and sacroiliac joint injections. With a piriformis injection, medication is injected into the piriformis muscle of your buttock. The sciatic nerve passes through or under this muscle. With a sacroiliac joint injection, medication is injected into an inflamed sacroiliac joint.

flamed sacroiliac joint (sacroiliitis). This pain can extend to the groin or down one or both legs and get worse when you sit for long periods, walk and run, or climb stairs.

A sacroiliac joint injection delivers medication into the area near the sacroiliac joint in order to soothe the inflamed joint, reduce swelling and relieve pain.

Piriformis muscle Your doctor may recommend a piriformis injection if your sciatic nerve is being pinched as it passes through the piriformis muscle, a muscle located behind the hip joint. This condition, known as piriformis syndrome, can cause an aching pain in the buttocks and more rarely in the hip, groin, buttock and tailbone, and back of the thigh.

A doctor may inject medication into your piriformis muscle to decrease inflammation, swelling and spasms and to soothe your irritated sciatic nerve. This procedure can help to reduce or relieve symptoms of pain and numbness.

Trigger point Trigger points are areas where your muscles and surrounding connective tissues are sensitive to touch. Trigger points are commonly located in the upper and lower back muscles. Pressure on these points can cause pain in the muscle and sometimes in seemingly unrelated parts of your body. This type of pain is known as myofascial pain. (To learn more about myofascial pain turn to page 38.)(To learn more about myofascial pain turn to page 38.)

If you're experiencing myofascial pain that hasn't responded to physical therapy or other conservative treatments, your doctor may suggest a trigger point injection. Injecting an anesthetic or a steroid directly into a trigger point may help reduce pain in the muscle, reduce inflammation or relax an overly sensitive muscle.

Effectiveness and safety

Injection therapy can provide significant relief from back and neck pain, but the injections don't help everyone. Research as to their effectiveness is ongoing. Keep in mind that it may take several injections for your doctor to locate the exact source of your pain. And if the injection is successful, it may still take up to two weeks for you to start experiencing pain relief.

Injection therapy is generally considered safe as long as steroid injections are limited to three or four a year. Temporary side effects may include soreness at the injection site, a red, flushed face, insomnia, a mild headache, dizziness, mood swings and a

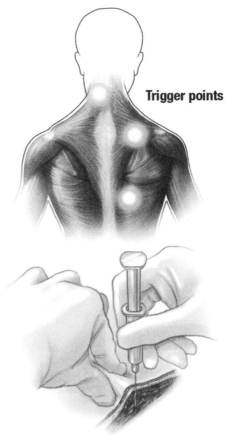

Trigger points

Injection into knotted muscle

Trigger point injection. A trigger point injection is designed to relieve back pain caused by small knots that can form in muscles or in tissues, leading to myofascial pain.

---

feeling of being revved up. If you have diabetes, you may experience a rise in your glucose levels.

Serious complications from injections don't happen often. They may include bleeding at the injection site, worsening numbness or pain, infection, or injury to a nerve.

RADIOFREQUENCY ABLATION

Radiofrequency ablation, also called radiofrequency denervation or neurotomy, uses heat generated by radio waves to target specific nerves and temporarily turn off their ability to send pain signals. Your doctor may recommend this procedure if your pain is confined to a facet joint that hasn't improved with conservative treatment.

To determine whether you might benefit from radiofrequency ablation, your doctor may first perform one or more medial branch blocks to pinpoint the exact site of your pain. A medial branch block involves injection of an anesthetic near the nerves (medial branch nerves) that supply a specific facet joint. These nerves carry pain signals from the joint to your brain. A medial branch block temporarily blocks the nerves from sending pain signals. If your pain is caused by the targeted facet joint, you may experience temporary pain relief. If the pain relief is significant, radiofrequency ablation at the same site may provide longer lasting relief.

Radiofrequency ablation usually is performed as an outpatient procedure. During the procedure, you may receive a mild sedative to calm you and help reduce any discomfort. You'll also receive an injection of anesthetic medication to numb nearby skin and tissues. Once the area is numb, your doctor inserts needles through your skin near the site of your pain to deliver radio waves to the targeted nerves. To guide the needles and make sure they're positioned properly, a doctor typically uses an X-ray

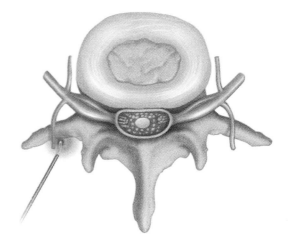

Radiofrequency ablation. This procedure uses heat generated from radio waves (see green shading) to stop a medial branch nerve from transmitting pain signals from an injured facet joint to the brain.

---

imaging procedure called fluoroscopy. He or she may also ask you questions about how you feel to ensure the needles are in the correct location.

Effectiveness and safety

Radiofrequency ablation isn't a permanent fix for back or neck pain, but it can make a difference for some people. You may experience modest, short-term pain relief or you might feel better for six months or longer. Sometimes, the treatment doesn't improve pain or function at all. If the procedure successfully reduces your pain, your doctor may recommend repeating it when the pain returns.

Common side effects of radiofrequency ablation may include numbness or pain at the injection site. You may also experience temporary weakness. Rarely, more serious complications may occur, including infection at the injection site, nerve damage, and long-term weakness or paralysis of the neck, back, arm or legs.

NERVE STIMULATION

Electrical nerve stimulation can sometimes reduce or relieve pain by sending electrical impulses to nerve pathways near a painful area in your neck or back. Exactly how the electrical stimulation works isn't fully understood, but medical scientists believe that electrical impulses disrupt pain sensations passing through the spinal cord. Electrical stimulation is also thought to trigger the nervous system to produce substances called enkephalins and endorphins that naturally reduce pain.

One type of nerve stimulation involves a surgically implanted spinal cord stimulator (see page 169). A commonly used nonsurgical stimulation therapy for back and neck conditions is called transcutaneous electrical nerve stimulation (TENS). TENS therapy uses a portable battery-powered device that's about the size of a deck of cards. Attached to the unit are electrodes that are connected by wires and that stick to your skin. The electrodes deliver low-level, painless electrical impulses that stimulate underlying nerves and cause a mild tingling sensation.

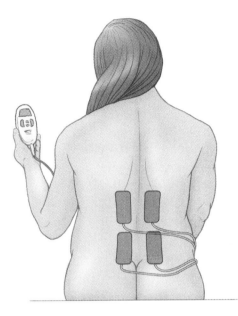

Transcutaneous electrical nerve stimulation (TENS). During TENS therapy, electrodes deliver electrical impulses to nearby nerve pathways, which can help control or relieve some types of pain.

If your doctor recommends TENS treatment, he or she may perform the therapy during office visits, refer you to a physical therapist who will perform the therapy or prescribe a TENS device you can use at home. You can also purchase less powerful over-the-counter TENS devices on your own.

If you're prescribed a device for home use, make sure you're fully instructed on how to use it, where to place the electrodes and what settings might be best for you. Medical staff can also help you determine how many times a day to use the device and for how long.

Effectiveness and safety

Studies show mixed results when it comes to the effectiveness of the therapy. While TENS appears to reduce pain and improve mobility in some people with back or neck problems, other people experience little or no benefit.

The device itself is safe for most people and won't give an electric shock. Some people develop skin irritation or a skin rash (contact dermatitis) from the electrode adhesive. TENS isn't recommended if you have an older pacemaker or an irregular heartbeat (heart arrhythmia) or if you're in the first trimester of a pregnancy.

TRACTION

Traction involves gently drawing the bones of the spine apart lengthwise in order to open up more space between them. In theory, traction takes pressure off nerve roots and disks in your spine.

A physical therapist most commonly performs traction, but chiropractors or other health care providers may also perform this treatment. During a traction session, you lie on a padded table while a health care provider gently applies a constant or intermittent stretching force to your neck or lower back.

A provider may perform this treatment using a mechanical traction device or his or her hands. Another traction technique is inversion therapy, which takes advantage of gravity by placing your body in a head-down position.

Effectiveness and safety

Research suggests that traction is less effective for back and neck pain than are other treatments. While some people may experience pain relief, it often tends to be short-lived. For this reason, traction isn't as common as it once was and your doctor or physical therapist may be less likely to recommend it.

While traction is generally considered safe, it's not advised if you're pregnant or you have certain health conditions, including osteoporosis, inflammatory arthritis, uncontrolled high blood pressure or heart disease.

MEDICATION

Medication can play a role in helping to reduce your pain if the pain is keeping you from staying active or from fully engaging in physical therapy. When possible, it's best to use over-the-counter medications (see Chapter 6 for a list of nonprescription options). Sometimes, however, nonprescription drugs don't provide adequate pain relief. In such instances, a doctor may prescribe one or more of the following medications.

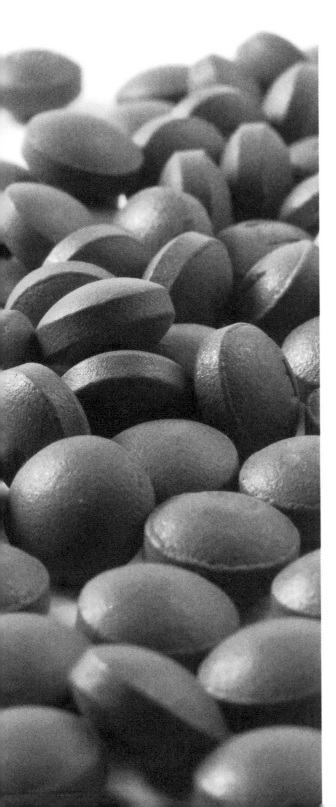

Nonsteroidal anti-inflammatory drugs (NSAIDs)

Prescription NSAIDs such as naproxen (Anaprox DS, Naprelan), diclofenac (Cataflam, Solaraze, others) and celecoxib (Celebrex) can help reduce back and neck pain during the first weeks of a painful episode or a flare-up of severe pain.

It's important to take only the dose you need for as short an amount of time as possible. Overuse of NSAIDs can cause serious side effects, including nausea, stomach pain, and stomach bleeding and ulcers. Large doses may also lead to kidney problems and high blood pressure and may increase your risk of heart attack and stroke.

Your doctor may recommend you take a prescription-strength NSAID for one or two weeks and then slowly taper off the medication as your body begins to recover and your pain decreases. If your pain doesn't diminish after several weeks on a prescription NSAID, consider discussing other treatment options with your doctor.

Muscle relaxants

Short-term use of muscle relaxants — such as cyclobenzaprine (Amrix) or tizanidine (Zanaflex) — may help get you through a brief bout of back or neck pain. Research indicates that while muscle relaxants reduce short-term pain for some people, they're not a proven therapy for chronic pain. These medications may also not be as effective for back and neck conditions as are NSAIDs. In some cases, your doctor may prescribe a muscle relaxant in addition to an NSAID.

Because the most common side effects of muscle relaxants are drowsiness and dizziness, your doctor may recommend that you take the medication before bed. If you take muscle relaxants during the day, you should avoid driving or operating heavy machinery. The sedating effect of muscle relaxants may be especially strong if you're an older adult.

Antidepressants

Although not specifically intended to treat back and neck conditions, low doses of certain antidepressants may reduce your pain, even when depression isn't a factor. The painkilling mechanism of these drugs still isn't fully understood. Antidepressants may increase neurotransmitters in the spinal cord that reduce pain signals.

Several types of antidepressants are used to treat back and neck pain. Serotonin and norepinephrine reuptake inhibitors (SNRIs) are one type and include the medications duloxetine (Cymbalta, Drizalma Sprinkle) and venlafaxine (Effexor XR). Tricyclic antidepressants — including amitriptyline, nortriptyline (Pamelor) and desipramine (Norpramin) — are another type of antidepressant that may provide some pain relief.

While these medications can be helpful for back and neck pain, some people find that the side effects outweigh the benefits. Common side effects of duloxetine include nausea, constipation, diarrhea, dry mouth, insomnia or excessive sweating. Venlafaxine can cause problems such as insomnia, weight loss or elevated blood pressure, and may worsen heart problems. Among the most common side effects of tricyclic antidepressants are dry mouth, constipation, dizziness and drowsiness.

Opioids

You've probably heard a lot about opioids — that they can treat pain but that this pain relief often comes at a high cost. The truth is that opioids are highly addictive, and the United States has witnessed an alarming increase in drug overdoses as a result of opioid medications.

Experts agree that opioids should only be considered for back and neck pain if the pain is severe, if other treatments haven't been effective, and if there's a low risk of misuse or addiction.

Experts also recommend that opioids be used at the lowest dose possible for the shortest time possible to help someone manage a brief episode of pain. Opioids are not recommended for the long-term treatment of chronic back and neck pain.

Common side effects of opioids include nausea, constipation, drowsiness, dizziness and itchy skin. Long-term use of the drugs carries many more serious risks. Ironically, one risk is that your sensitivity to pain might increase. Some people who take opioids for pain develop what's called hyperalgesia. With this condition, your body becomes more sensitive to pain and feels pain more intensely, the exact opposite of what taking a pain medication is meant to achieve.

Another common problem is that you may develop a tolerance to the opioid over time. This means that your body gets used to the dose of opioids that you're taking, leading you to increase your dose over and over again to achieve the same level of pain relief you've come to expect.

Addiction is a risk even if you take an opioid as prescribed. It's a risk even if you don't have a history of unhealthy substance use or mental illness, both of which can make addiction more likely.

Addiction is more common if you take opioids for long periods of time, but you're still at risk of addiction even if you take opioids only for a short time. Researchers have found that taking opioid medications for short-term back pain increases your risk of long-term use, which in turn increases your risk of addiction.

Before you consider taking opioids for your condition, make sure to talk to your doctor about other treatments and medications. Studies show that NSAIDs and antidepressants can be as effective as opioids in reducing back and neck pain, and without the same risks.

Tramadol

Tramadol (ConZip, Ultram) is a pain-relieving drug with opioid-like properties. It can be a last-resort option for chronic pain that's not responding to other measures, or for temporary use with a flare-up of pain.

The risk of side effects with tramadol, including constipation, drowsiness and dry mouth, is generally lower than with opioids. Although the risk of addiction is also less than with opioids, when tramadol is used for a long time it may become habit-forming, causing mental or physical dependence. For this reason, your doctor will likely recommend a low dose for the shortest period possible

STEM CELL TREATMENTS

Medical scientists are constantly working on emerging treatments to treat back and neck pain. One such treatment uses stem cells — cells from which all other cells with specialized functions are generated. Researchers are studying whether stem cells taken from your bone marrow (mesenchymal stem cells) and injected into a damaged spinal disk might help to repair that disk.

A spinal disk has a soft, jellylike center called the nucleus. As you age, the nucleus loses water content and height, providing less cushioning for your spine. Early research suggests that injecting stem cells into a damaged disk may be a safe, effective way to at least partly regenerate and rehydrate damaged disks, reducing pain and improving quality of life.

An added benefit is that stem cell therapy appears to be less invasive than surgery. But the research is still in its initial stages, and more study is needed to determine if stem cell therapy is a viable treatment option for back and neck pain.

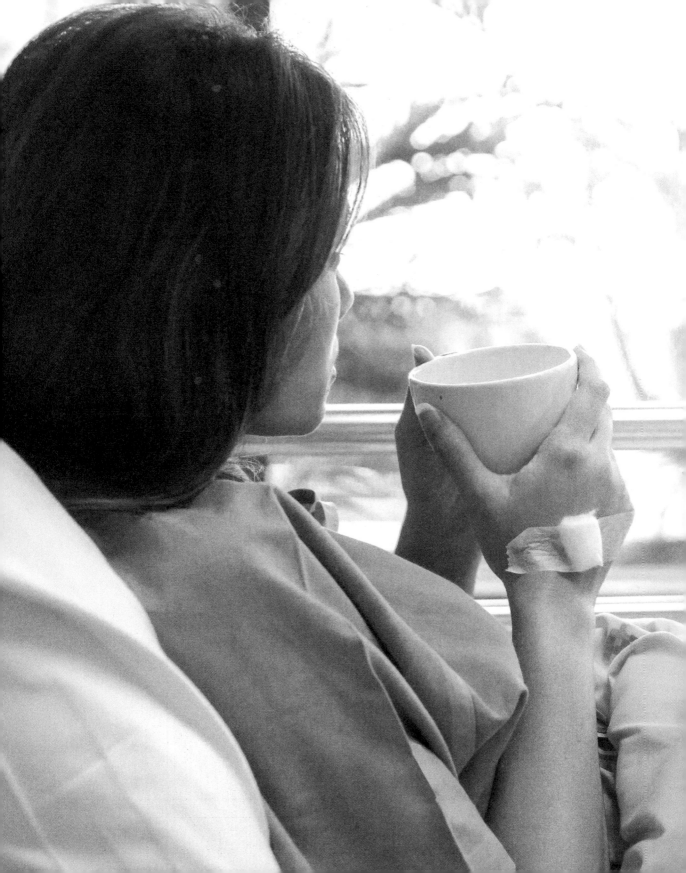

CHAPTER 9

Surgery

If your back or neck condition is causing you severe pain that won't go away, you might have turned directly to this chapter in the belief that surgery is your best option. The truth is that while back and neck surgery can help treat some causes of pain, it's often not necessary.

Back and neck problems typically respond to nonsurgical treatments, such as physical therapy, injection therapy or medication. If other treatments haven't been successful and your pain remains persistent and debilitating, surgery may be an option.

Surgery for most back and neck conditions is elective. This means that while surgery may be helpful, your situation is not an emergency. Elective surgery doesn't need to be performed urgently or within a specific time period. A doctor may recommend im-

mediate surgery in rare cases when a spinal condition is life-threatening or could cause permanent damage, such as paralysis.

Surgery may help to reduce or relieve pain located in an area of your neck or back. More often, it relieves pain or numbness that goes down one or both arms or legs due to a pinched (compressed) nerve. Nerves can become compressed due to degenerative changes in the bones (vertebrae) and disks of the spine. These changes can also lead to a variety of other painful back and neck problems. Additional conditions that may warrant surgery include spinal tumors and spine deformities.

It's important to know that while surgery may improve how you feel, it might not eliminate all of your pain. In addition, surgery doesn't cure diseases such as arthritis, nor does it guarantee you won't experience back or neck problems in the future.

When it comes to back and neck pain, surgery is often a treatment of last resort. But if your pain has been keeping you on the sidelines for too long and no other treatment seems to be working, surgery may help relieve your symptoms and improve your ability to engage in and enjoy daily life.

SURGERY BASICS

Before we discuss the surgeries most commonly used to treat back and neck conditions, it may be helpful to have some basic information about surgical terms your doctor or surgeon may be using that are unfamiliar to you. Following are some explanations that may help you better understand how back and neck surgery is performed.

Anterior vs. posterior vs. lateral

During back and neck surgery, a surgeon may access the problem area through an incision in the front (anterior), back (posterior) or side (lateral) of the body.

Anterior approach During this procedure, you lie on your back. Your surgeon makes an incision in your throat or abdomen to gain access to the front of your spine.

Posterior approach For this surgical approach, you lie facedown. Your surgeon makes an incision in your neck or your back to gain access to the back of your spine. The

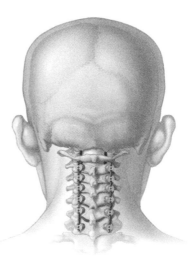

Anterior approach   **Posterior approach**

Anterior vs. posterior. Surgery on the spine may be performed by accessing the spine from the front (anterior approach) or from the back (posterior approach).

incision may be directly over your spine or on either side of your spine.

Lateral approach With this type of surgery, you lie on your side so that your doctor can make an incision down the side of your body. The lateral approach is less common than the posterior and anterior approaches.

Open vs. minimally invasive

Surgery involving your spine may be performed using traditional open surgery that may involve a large incision or using minimally invasive techniques with smaller incisions. Which approach your surgeon recommends is generally dependent on the specifics of your particular case.

Open surgery During open spine surgery, you typically receive general anesthesia, meaning you're asleep, or unconscious, during the surgery. Your surgeon makes a large incision and moves muscle and other soft tissue aside to reach the spine.

Minimally invasive surgery This type of surgery most often uses either general anesthesia or regional anesthesia, which numbs a region of your body while you're kept awake or lightly sedated. The surgeon makes one or more small incisions without moving muscle or other soft tissue.

A typical minimally invasive method uses a tube-shaped metal tool called a tubular retractor. The surgeon inserts the retractor through the small incision to reach the spinal

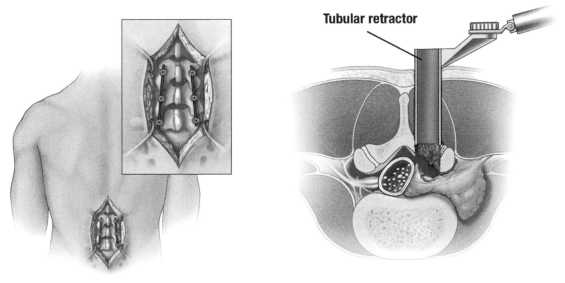

Open surgery

Minimally invasive surgery

Open vs. minimally invasive. With open surgery a large incision is made to gain access to the spine. Minimally invasive surgery accesses the spine by way of one or more small incisions.

column. The retractor holds open your muscle while the surgeon inserts surgical instruments through the retractor to perform the surgery. Hardware such as screws, rods or plates also may fit through the retractor.

Minimally invasive surgery may also involve use of an endoscope, a flexible tube with a light and camera used to look deep into the body. Minimally invasive surgery usually results in less bleeding, a shorter hospital stay and a faster recovery. Often, the procedure can be performed on an outpatient basis, meaning you return home the same day. Not everyone qualifies for minimally invasive surgery, and the decision is best made by you and your doctor.

DECOMPRESSION SURGERY

Surgery that's performed to relieve pressure on one or more nerves in your spine is called decompression surgery. It involves removing a portion of bone or soft tissue that's pushing on (compressing) the spinal cord, a spinal nerve root or both.

Decompression surgery helps alleviate pressure on compressed nerves by giving them more space. In addition to reducing pain, decompression surgery may relieve numbness, tingling and weakness affecting one or both arms or legs.

Nerve compression is often associated with bony overgrowths (bone spurs) that develop on the spinal column. Bone spurs are often linked to degeneration of spinal verte-brae from years of wear and tear and diseases such as osteoarthritis. A bone spur may narrow the spinal canal — the hollow passageway within the spine through which your spinal cord and nerves run from your brain to your pelvis — and pinch the cord or nearby nerve roots. The medical term for narrowing of the spinal canal is spinal stenosis.

Nerve compression may also result from a ruptured (herniated) disk. Disks, located between the bones of your spine, contain a gel-like material in their centers. Sometimes, this soft center can push out through a crack in a disk's tough exterior and place pressure on the spinal cord or nearby nerve roots.

To treat a compressed nerve, your surgeon may perform decompression surgery. Decompression surgery may be done by itself or in combination with another surgery, such as fusion surgery. (See page 154 for more about fusion surgery.)

Why it may be done

Your doctor may recommend decompression surgery if other treatments have failed to relieve disabling or worsening symptoms caused by a compressed nerve. This type of surgery may be helpful if your symptoms are associated with:
- Spinal stenosis
- A herniated disk
- Shifting of a vertebra, causing malalignment with the vertebra above or below it (spondylolisthesis)

- A fluid-filled growth in a joint (synovial cyst)
- A spinal fracture or tumor

Rarely, in case of severe nerve compression that may be life-threatening or result in permanent nerve damage, such as cauda equina syndrome, decompression surgery may need to be performed urgently.

How it's done

Decompression surgery may be performed as an open procedure or a minimally invasive procedure (see page 151). During the surgery, you may lie on your chest, back or side. A surgeon makes one or more incisions at the site of the nerve compression and removes bone or soft tissue compressing nearby nerves. Your surgeon may use an X-ray imaging procedure (fluoroscopy) that allows him or her to view your spinal column during surgery.

Types of decompression surgery

The most common types of decompression surgery involve removing either vertebral bone or damaged disk tissue, or both.

Bone removal Bone removal can help to relieve pressure on the spinal cord or spinal nerve roots by enlarging your spinal canal. Surgeries to remove bone include:
- **Laminectomy.** This procedure creates space for spinal nerves by removing some or all of the back part of a vertebra that covers your spinal canal, known as the lamina.
- **Laminotomy.** Only a portion of the lamina is removed, typically by carving a hole just big enough to relieve the pressure in a particular spot.
- **Laminoplasty.** This surgery is performed only on vertebrae in the neck (cervical spine). It enlarges the space within the spinal canal by "hinging open" the lamina. A surgeon implants metal hardware to hold the lamina open.
- **Foraminotomy.** It relieves pressure by widening the bony opening (foramen) through which a nerve root exits the spinal column.
- **Corpectomy.** A surgeon removes the front part of a vertebra, often in preparation for fusion surgery. The disk above or below the vertebra also may be removed.
- **Facetectomy.** This surgery removes one or more of the small joints (facet joints) located at each vertebral level of the spine. A facetectomy is often combined with fusion surgery.

Disk removal Decompression surgery may remove some or all of a damaged disk. Ideally, just the portion of the disk that's pinching the nerve is removed, relieving the pressure but leaving most of the disk intact. If your entire disk must be taken out, your surgeon may need to perform other procedures to support and stabilize that section of the spine.

Surgeries to remove spinal disks include:
- **Diskectomy.** This procedure, performed with open surgery, removes some or all

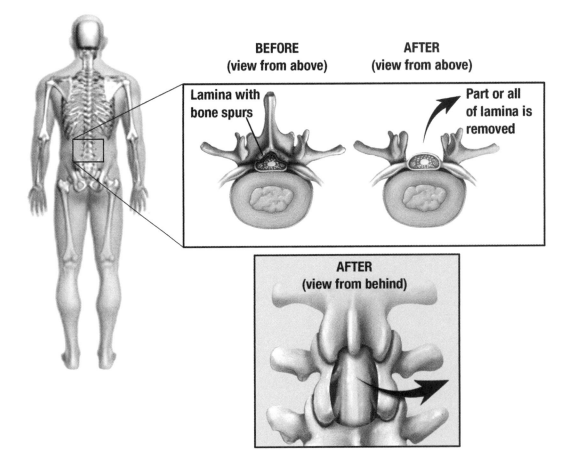

BEFORE
(view from above)

AFTER
(view from above)

Lamina with bone spurs

Part or all of lamina is removed

AFTER
(view from behind)

Laminectomy. Laminectomy is surgery that relieves compression on spinal nerves and creates space by removing the lamina — the back part of a vertebra that covers your spinal canal.

of a damaged disk that is pressing on nearby nerves.

- **Microdiskectomy.** It's the most common decompression procedure for removing disk tissue. Microdiskectomy involves the use of a high-powered microscope to view the disk being removed. The surgery can be done using an open or a minimally invasive approach.
- **Endoscopic diskectomy.** In this minimally invasive surgery, your surgeon inserts a long tube with a video camera attached (endoscope) through a small incision. This tiny camera allows the surgeon to closely view the damaged disk during surgery.

SPINAL FUSION SURGERY

Spinal fusion surgery, also known as stabilization surgery, permanently connects two

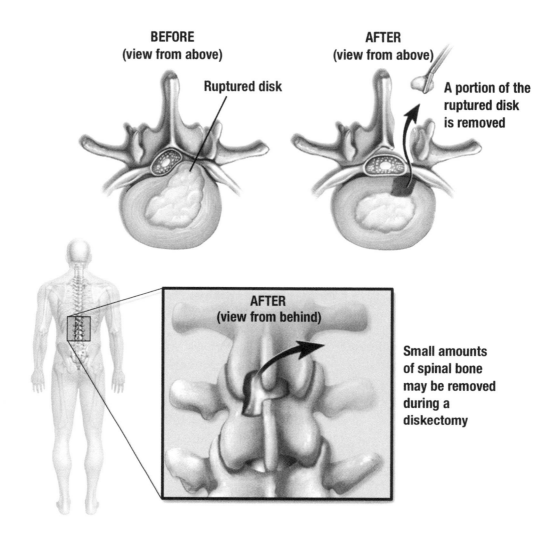

BEFORE
(view from above)

Ruptured disk

AFTER
(view from above)

A portion of the
ruptured disk
is removed

AFTER
(view from behind)

Small amounts
of spinal bone
may be removed
during a
diskectomy

Diskectomy. Diskectomy is a surgical procedure to remove the damaged portion of a herniated disk in your spine. A herniated disk can irritate or compress nearby nerves.

or more vertebrae in your spine, eliminating painful movement between the vertebrae and stabilizing your spine. By stopping movement in certain locations of your back or neck, fusion surgery may reduce your symptoms. Spinal fusion surgery may also be performed to help correct a deformity.

While spinal fusion can be helpful for some people, immobilizing a section of the spine places additional stress and strain on nearby sections. This may lead to adjacent segment disease — a condition in which degeneration develops in the bones of the spine above and below the fused bones.

This condition can sometimes cause new pain to develop, so you may need additional spine surgery in the future.

Why it may be done

Your doctor may recommend fusion surgery if other treatments haven't helped relieve chronic back or neck pain and if the pain is severe enough to significantly limit your ability to function on a daily basis. A surgeon may also fuse two or more vertebrae to stabilize your spine after major decompression surgery.

Spinal fusion may be recommended if your symptoms are associated with:

- Spinal weakness or instability due to abnormal or excessive motion between two vertebrae
- Spondylolisthesis
- A recurrent herniated disk
- Spinal cord compression myelopathy
- A synovial cyst
- A spinal fracture
- Deformities of the spine, such as scoliosis (see page 52)

How it's done

Spinal fusion surgery may be performed as an open or a minimally invasive procedure (see page 151). During the surgery, you may lie on your back, stomach or side while your surgeon makes one or more incisions to gain access to your spine. To view your spinal column during surgery, your surgeon may use an X-ray imaging procedure called fluoroscopy.

Fusion surgery involves techniques designed to mimic the normal healing process of broken bones. During the procedure, your surgeon implants a bone graft within the space between two spinal vertebrae. The bone graft may be some of your own bone (autograft) — most often taken from your pelvis — or it may come from a bone bank (allograft). In selected cases, some surgeons use artificial bone.

The bone graft acts like glue to fuse the vertebrae together. Your surgeon may also use metal plates, screws and rods to hold the vertebrae together so that they can heal into one solid unit. Typically the vertebrae start to fuse in three to six months. But it could take up to a full year for the area to completely heal.

Types of fusion surgery

Surgeons use a variety of surgical approaches and techniques to fuse the spine. Depending on your back or neck condition, your doctor may discuss one or more of these approaches:

Anterior cervical diskectomy and fusion (ACDF) During an ACDF, your surgeon makes an incision in the front of your neck. He or she then removes the damaged disk tissue between two vertebrae before fusing the bones together. ACDF is the most common type of fusion for the neck.

MY DOCTOR IS RECOMMENDING SURGERY. SHOULD I GET A SECOND OPINION?

If a spine surgeon is recommending elective surgery to reduce your symptoms and you feel confident in both the plan and your surgeon, you don't necessarily need a second opinion.

On the other hand, if you'd like to gather more information or if you're not fully comfortable with your surgeon's recommendation, getting a second or third opinion can be a sensible approach. Spine surgeons may hold different opinions about when to operate, what type of surgery to perform and whether surgery is warranted at all. By becoming thoroughly informed about your condition, available treatment options and possible outcomes, you'll feel more confident about making a decision.

You can ask your surgeon to recommend another spine specialist to consult for a second opinion. If you don't have a recommendation, look for spine specialists who have experience delivering high-quality care and outcomes. Recommendations of friends and family members, or former patients, can be helpful as well.

Plan to bring your medical records, including copies of all tests, scans, exams and previous treatments, with you to the appointment. Be clear about what you're looking for from the second opinion. Do you need confirmation that your current treatment recommendation is the best approach for you? Or are you looking for other options?

If the second doctor has a different opinion than the first, you may want to talk more about your condition with your first doctor. Or you might prefer to seek another opinion from a third doctor.

A second or third opinion can give you extra confidence that you're doing the best thing. You may choose to continue with your first doctor. If you decide to transfer your care to another doctor, make sure that you communicate this to your original doctor.

SURGERY ENHANCEMENTS

Technological advancements continue to help improve spinal surgery outcomes. Enhancements to surgery include:

Image-guided surgery

Many surgeons now use image guidance during surgery to help ensure precise placement of screws into vertebrae. Image-guidance technology allows a surgeon to see in real time exactly where a screw is going as it is anchored into bone. This significantly reduces the risk of a screw being positioned in a less than ideal location (malposition).

Robot-guided surgery

A relatively new fusion technique involves the use of a robot in the operating room. The robotic system guides a robotic arm to a predetermined position during fusion surgery. Under the guidance of a surgeon, the robotic arm inserts stabilizing screws into vertebrae at precise locations on the spine. This precision helps to reduce the risk that you'll need additional surgery to reposition incorrectly placed screws. In the future, robotic guidance may be used in other types of spinal surgery as well.

Posterior cervical or lumbar fusion In this procedure, your surgeon makes an incision down the back of your neck (cervical) or middle of your back (lumbar) to remove damaged disk bone and tissue and fuse two or more bones together.

Lumbar interbody fusion During this back surgery, a surgeon removes the damaged disk and implants a spacer, called an interbody cage, between your vertebrae. The cage holds the bones apart the way a disk does. This device is usually made of surgical-grade metal or plastic and often contains crushed bone.

There are several types of lumbar interbody fusion methods, including:

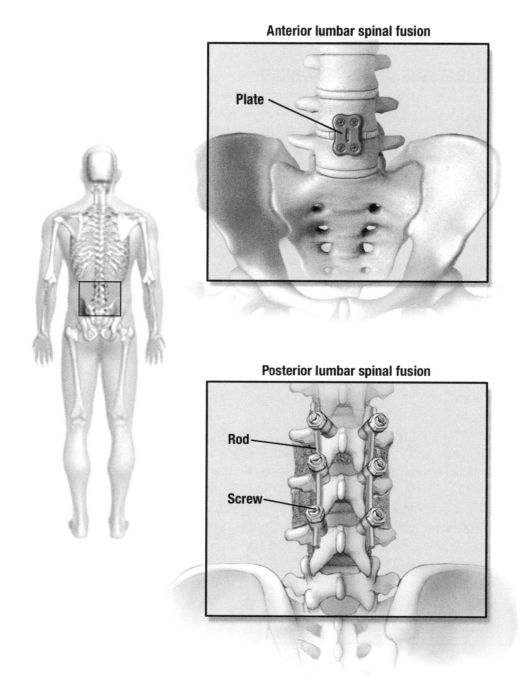

Anterior lumbar spinal fusion

Plate

Posterior lumbar spinal fusion

Rod

Screw

Spinal fusion surgery. Spinal fusion is surgery to permanently connect two or more vertebrae in your spine, eliminating motion between them. Metal plates, screws and rods may be used to hold the vertebrae together.

COMPLICATIONS OF SPINE SURGERY

Research shows that your risk of problems (complications) related to spine surgery are lower when a highly experienced surgeon performs the procedure. Risks of spine surgery include, but may not be limited to, the following:

- Excessive bleeding
- Infection
- Blood clots
- Allergic reaction to anesthesia
- Problems with healing
- Further nerve damage or spinal cord injury
- Implant malfunction (rod, screw, plate, or artificial disk or joint)
- A tear in the tough, outermost membrane around the spinal cord (dura)
- Injuries to structures in the throat during neck surgery, including the voice box
- Paralysis or death (rare)

Keep in mind that every person is different, and your risk of complications may be different from that of someone else having the same surgery. In general, your risks depend on:

- Your overall medical condition
- Which area or areas of the spine are being operated on
- Whether the surgeon is using an anterior, posterior or lateral surgical approach
- Whether you've had previous surgery in the same area
- Whether you have chronic health problems, such as a weak immune system, a history of infection, obesity, diabetes, rheumatoid arthritis, alcoholism or smoking

For information about your risks and possible complications, talk to your doctor.

- **Posterior lumbar interbody fusion (PLIF).** In this procedure, a surgeon gains access to your spine with an incision in your back. He or she performs a laminec- tomy to reach and remove the damaged disk before performing interbody fusion.
- **Transforaminal lumbar interbody fusion (TLIF).** This surgery is similar to

PLIF, but it involves both a laminectomy and a facetectomy.

- **Anterior lumbar interbody fusion (ALIF).** A surgeon gains access to your spine by making an incision in your abdomen, usually with the help of a vascular surgeon. He or she removes the damaged disk in preparation for interbody fusion.
- **Lateral lumbar interbody fusion.** Your surgeon makes an incision down your side to access the spine and perform interbody fusion.

TUMOR SURGERY

If you have a tumor or other abnormal growth (lesion) on your spine, your doctor may recommend surgery to remove it. Spinal tumors may affect the bones of the spine, or they may begin within the spinal cord or the covering of the spinal cord (dura). Spinal tumors can be noncancerous (benign) or cancerous (malignant).

When a tumor presses on the spinal cord or nearby nerve roots, it can cause symptoms such as numbness, muscle weakness and loss of muscle control. As the tumor grows, it may cause pain, vertebral fractures or spinal instability. In some instances, a tumor can be life-threatening and cause permanent disability or paralysis.

Why it may be done

Surgery is often the treatment of choice for problematic tumors that can be removed without significant risk of spinal cord or nerve injury. Your doctor may recommend surgery if your tumor is malignant or if it's causing severe problems, such as pain, bone fractures or harmful nerve compression. Sometimes your surgeon may not be able to remove all of the tumor. If the tumor is malignant, your doctor may recommend radiation therapy, chemotherapy or both.

How it's done

During surgery to remove a tumor, you typically lie on your chest or back while a surgeon makes an incision at the site of the tumor. The surgeon may remove some vertebral bone in an effort to remove the tumor or gain access to it within the spinal cord or dura. If needed, two or more vertebrae may be fused together to stabilize your spine after removing the tumor.

Newer techniques and instruments allow surgeons to reach tumors that were once considered inaccessible. Sometimes, surgeons may use a high-powered microscope or endoscope (microsurgery) to make it easier to distinguish a tumor from healthy tissue. Doctors can also monitor the function of the spinal cord and other important nerves during surgery to minimize the chance that they'll be injured.

SPINAL DEFORMITY SURGERY

If you have a severe spinal deformity that affects the alignment of your spine, your doctor may recommend surgery. A common spinal deformity is scoliosis, a sideways curvature of the spine (see page 53). People most often develop scoliosis in childhood or adolescence, but some adults develop a condition called degenerative scoliosis, usually around age 65 or older. In certain cases, a misaligned spine can lead to back pain and the compression of nearby nerves.

In childhood, surgery for scoliosis is performed to improve spinal alignment and help prevent the abnormal curvature from worsening as a child grows. In adulthood, surgery can help to straighten the spine and open up space to relieve nerve compression.

Why it may be done

Most of the time, surgery isn't necessary to correct an abnormal curvature of the spine, but a doctor may recommend surgery for:
- Children or adolescents who have severe scoliosis or whose abnormal spinal curvature is likely to become severe over time
- Adults with severe degenerative scoliosis who continue to experience significant and worsening pain and weakness despite undergoing nonsurgical treatments

How it's done

The most common type of surgery to treat scoliosis is spinal fusion. By fusing two or more vertebrae together, surgery can help to better align an abnormally curved spine.

Your surgeon may use an anterior approach, posterior approach or both to perform the fusion. The surgery may be open or minimally invasive (see page 151).

MOTION PRESERVATION SURGERY

In recent years, motion preservation surgeries have emerged as an alternative to spinal fusion. These surgeries aim to reduce severe pain and maintain your spine's stability while preserving natural movement in the affected area. By allowing your spine to maintain its mobility, motion preservation surgeries may help lower the risk of adjacent segment disease, which can occur after fusion surgery.

Currently, two emerging procedures aim to reduce pain while preserving spinal motion.

Disk replacement surgery

Disk replacement surgery removes a damaged disk and implants an artificial disk between the two vertebrae. This surgery may be performed in the back or neck. When the surgery is performed in the neck, it's often called cervical disk arthroplasty.

Disk replacement helps to relieve nerve pain in your arms or legs and maintain spinal motion and stability. Sometimes a surgeon may perform disk replacement surgery with spinal fusion. The artificial disk helps your spine remain as flexible as possible in the fused area.

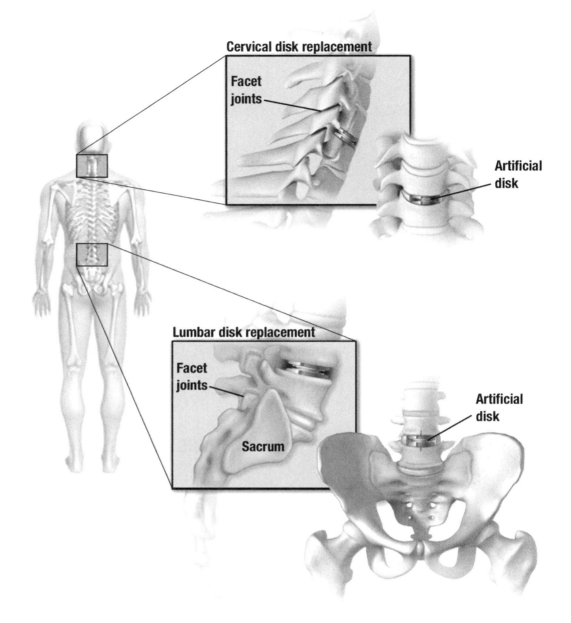

Cervical disk replacement

Facet joints

Artificial disk

Lumbar disk replacement

Facet joints

Sacrum

Artificial disk

Disk replacement surgery. This surgery is a newer procedure that replaces a problem disk with an artificial one made of metal and plastic. An artificial disk helps maintain spinal flexibility.

Artificial disks are usually made of a curved top and bottom metal plate. The top plate attaches to the vertebra above the removed disk while the bottom plate is secured to the vertebra below the disk. These smooth plates slide across each other to allow for spinal motion. Some artificial disks contain a soft, plastic-like center between the plates to cushion the spine and absorb shock.

Disk replacement surgery isn't appropriate for everyone. It's recommended for healthy adults, generally those younger in age, who have stable spines and who haven't responded to more conservative treatments for a herniated or damaged disk. Disk replacement surgery generally isn't recommended for people with advanced osteoarthritis of the facet joints, weakened bones due to osteopenia or osteoporosis, spinal deformities, or destabilizing spine conditions such as spondylolisthesis or inflammatory arthritis (ankylosing spondylitis).

Because disk replacement is a relatively new surgery, research into its long-term effectiveness is ongoing. Some studies suggest that disk replacement surgery may have fewer complications when performed in the neck compared with the back. For some people, disk replacement in the neck may be more effective than a diskectomy with spinal fusion.

Facet replacement surgery

If your surgeon must remove a significant portion of your facet joint during decompression surgery, he or she typically stabilizes the joint by performing fusion surgery. Facet replacement surgery allows a surgeon to replace part or all of a damaged facet joint with an artificial joint. This helps to preserve the joint's natural motion and decrease the risk of damage to the spine above and below the joint.

A surgeon may replace a facet joint to relieve severe and chronic pain caused by a worn facet joint (facet joint disease), spinal stenosis or stenosis with spondylolisthesis. The artificial joint is made of surgical-grade metal, plastic-like materials or a combination of the two.

Facet replacement surgery is still in the experimental stages and is less commonly performed than other spinal surgeries. Researchers continue to study its effectiveness and risks.

LIMITATIONS AFTER SURGERY

In the days and weeks after surgery, some activities will help you heal while others should be avoided. Your surgical team will likely recommend that you walk several times a day, possibly with the use of a walker or other assistive device to help prevent falls. Depending on the type of surgery you have, you may be asked to wear a brace or neck collar.

Eating a healthy diet and taking a daily multivitamin also can help promote healing. If you don't get 1,000 to 1,500 mg of calcium with vitamin D in your daily diet, your doctor may suggest taking a supplement. Including high-fiber foods and drinking plenty of water can help you avoid constipation, which is a side effect of general anesthesia and opioid medications.

Common restrictions

Your doctor will discuss restrictions you should maintain following surgery. These limitations may last for weeks or months depending on the activity and the type of surgery performed. These are some common restrictions after spinal surgery:

Driving You shouldn't drive or use heavy machinery if you take prescription pain medication after surgery. Usually, people who wear a brace also are not allowed to drive. Depending on the type of surgery you have, your doctor may ask you to avoid driving for up to three months.

Alcohol If you take opioid pain medications after surgery, you'll need to avoid drinking alcohol. The same may be true for certain over-the-counter pain medications. If you have questions about your pain medications, talk to your pharmacist or doctor.

Tobacco products If you use tobacco products, your doctor will instruct you to stop using them well ahead of your surgery date. After surgery, you'll be asked to continue avoiding tobacco products until your bones are fully healed — sometimes up to a year or more.

Nicotine, carbon monoxide and other poisons in tobacco products increase the risk of complications after surgery. Examples of complications include poor bone and wound healing, pneumonia, blood clots, and high blood pressure. If you want help to quit smoking, talk to your doctor. There are many resources available that can help you.

Baths After surgery, you'll need to make sure you don't soak your surgical incision underwater, such as in a bath, hot tub, whirlpool or swimming pool. You may need to follow this restriction for at least four weeks or until your doctor gives you approval to submerge the incision in water.

Pain relievers Certain pain relievers can affect how your bones heal and how thin your blood is. Examples of include aspirin, aspirin-containing products, ibuprofen (Advil, Motrin IB) and naproxen sodium (Aleve). Be sure to talk with your doctor about what you can take for pain — especially if you already take blood-thinning medication.

Most people may take acetaminophen (Tylenol, others) as needed. However, taking too much acetaminophen can damage your liver. Talk to your doctor about how much of the medication you can safely take.

Heat Applying heat after surgery may make the surgical area swell. Your doctor or physical therapist may recommend using ice on your back or neck to reduce pain, stiffness and swelling.

Heavy lifting After surgery, avoid lifting objects weighing more than 5 to 10 pounds, unless your surgical team says it's OK to do so. When you do lift something, hold it close to your body and avoid lifting it above your head. (See page 180 for proper lifting techniques.)

Pushing and pulling Unless you get the OK from your doctor, don't push or pull objects greater than 5 to 10 pounds, such as a vacuum cleaner or grocery cart.

Bending, twisting or stooping Don't do anything that makes you bend, twist or stoop down. Examples include emptying the dishwasher, tying your shoes and trying to pick something up from the floor.

Exercise Avoid exercising until your doctor tells you it's safe to do so. Discuss with your doctor or a physical therapist which types of exercise are best.

CONTINUED PAIN

After back or neck surgery, it's normal to experience some pain or discomfort. You may feel pain in the area of the incision and aching in your neck, back, arm or leg as your nerves heal. Muscle spasms may also happen in these areas of your body.

Your pain and discomfort should start to diminish in the first few weeks after surgery. In time, you may feel little to no pain. Or you may continue to experience some pain, but at a noticeably lower level.

Causes of continued pain

Many people experience less pain and enjoy a higher quality of life after spine surgery. For some people, though, the pain doesn't improve or it gets worse. Other people notice a new pain.

Many factors may contribute to ongoing pain after surgery. Temporary complications from surgery might cause short-term pain that goes away on its own or gets better with conservative treatment. In some cases, the surgery may fail to address the true source of your pain — or fail to treat the problem fully. In other instances, an operation on the spine may cause a new problem to develop. Sometimes, there's no identifiable reason for continued pain after surgery.

People who undergo spinal surgery may experience continued pain for the following reasons:

Bleeding Sometimes after surgery, a build-up of blood (hematoma) forms under the skin, inside a muscle or in the epidural space. This can cause painful bruising and swelling. Usually the body reabsorbs the excess blood and the hematoma goes away on its own. If the hematoma doesn't heal, your doctor may need to surgically drain the excess blood.

Infection A common risk of any surgery is an infection. You could get an infection in a superficial wound, in a deep wound or near an implant (a disk, rod, screw or plate). An infection can cause increased tenderness, redness or swelling at the incision site. You may also develop a fever and notice drainage, bleeding or a bad odor coming from the incision. If you have any of these signs of infection after spine surgery, contact your doctor.

Deconditioning In some people, reduced muscle strength and endurance (deconditioning) can contribute to a painful recovery. The surgery itself may lead to muscle weakness, and you might compound the problem if you avoid physical activity out of fear that any movement will add to your discomfort. Exercises approved by your doctor or physical therapist can help to strengthen your muscles and relieve pain.

Spinal stenosis Sometimes decompression surgery fails to open up enough space in the spine to relieve a compressed nerve. Or you may develop adjacent segment disease after your surgery. This can cause your spine to narrow further, leading to nerve pain in an arm or leg.

Painful disks After diskectomy or fusion surgery, added stress to your spine may cause pain to develop in one or more disks near the site of the surgery.

Spinal instability Instability of the spine due to slippage of a vertebra (spondylolisthesis) may occur after spine surgery, especially if a large portion of bone is removed during decompression. Spondylolisthesis may also be a natural part of the aging process that happens regardless of whether you have surgery.

Pseudarthrosis Sometimes bones fail to fully heal or fuse after spine surgery. This condition is called pseudarthrosis. Pseudarthrosis doesn't always cause pain but it can lead to pain in some people. You're at greater risk of pseudarthrosis if you use tobacco products or steroids, take nonsteroidal anti-inflammatory medications (NSAIDs) after surgery, or have certain diseases, such as diabetes.

Disk herniation If surgery doesn't remove all of the disk tissue that's pressing on a nerve, you may continue to feel nerve pain. Or your surgeon may remove all of the damaged tissue, but the disk degenerates further and becomes herniated again.

Nerve damage Painful nerve damage can happen before or after surgery. In some cases, a severely compressed nerve may become permanently damaged. Decompression surgery relieves the pressure, but the damaged nerve continues to produce pain. On rare occasions, a nerve may be injured during surgery.

Spinal joint pain Sometimes a facet joint or sacroiliac joint is injured during surgery, resulting in joint pain. Adjacent segment disease also can cause a joint to deteriorate and become painful after surgery.

Preexisting conditions Some people begin to notice new symptoms after surgery in other parts of their spines or bodies. It's possible that this "new" pain was actually there before surgery, but a more painful area of your spine got more of your attention.

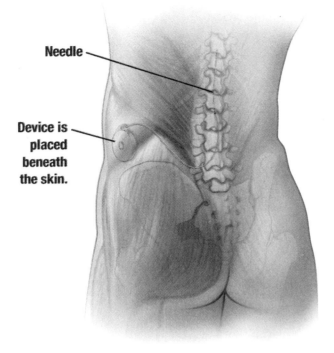

Needle

Device is placed beneath the skin.

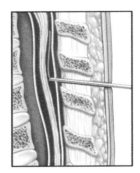

The needle is inserted into the fluid-filled space within the spinal canal.

Spinal cord stimulator. The device consists of a thin wire with an attached needle (electrode) and a small, pacemaker-like battery pack (generator). During a surgical procedure, the electrode is placed within the spinal canal and the generator is placed under the skin.

For example, a specific joint or disk might have been contributing to your pain. When surgery relieved pain in a different area, this other source of pain became easier to notice. This is called masked or hidden pain.

FAILED BACK SURGERY SYNDROME

It's disappointing when surgery doesn't treat your pain the way you'd hoped it would.

Sometimes the disappointment stems from unrealistic expectations. While spinal surgery may help relieve your symptoms and improve your daily functioning, it may not completely eliminate all of your pain. Having realistic expectations and a positive outlook can help you make the most of your surgery.

In other instances, surgery fails to meet the realistic expectations of both the patient and the surgeon. This situation is often called failed back surgery syndrome (FBSS). Accurate estimates of FBSS are hard to come by, but it's thought that potentially 10% of people who undergo spinal surgery experience this outcome.

If your doctor can identify the cause of your continued pain, physical therapy and other nonsurgical treatments may be able to treat the problem. Depending on your condition, additional surgery may be another option.

Spinal cord stimulator

If there's no clear cause for your continued pain after surgery, or if conservative treatments for a known cause aren't successful, your doctor may suggest a spinal cord stimulator. This surgically implanted device delivers low-level electrical pulses to nerves in the spinal cord.

Exactly how electrical stimulation works isn't fully understood, but medical scientists believe electrical impulses may override pain signals passing through the spinal cord.

During implantation, a surgeon places a wire within the spinal canal. The wire is connected to a small electrical generator (stimulator) implanted beneath the skin. A hand-held remote control allows you to operate the spinal cord stimulator as needed to manage your pain.

Before implanting a spinal cord stimulator, your doctor will first perform a test to make sure the device will help you and ensure that it's properly placed. The test involves placing wires with electrodes in your spine to mimic a spinal cord stimulator. The electrical generator remains outside your body during this trial run. If the trial provides significant pain relief, your doctor will perform surgery to implant the spinal cord stimulator.

A spinal cord stimulator successfully reduces pain in some people and is considered safe. Complications include device malfunction and infection. Very rarely, a life-threatening hematoma may form in the epidural space and must be surgically drained.

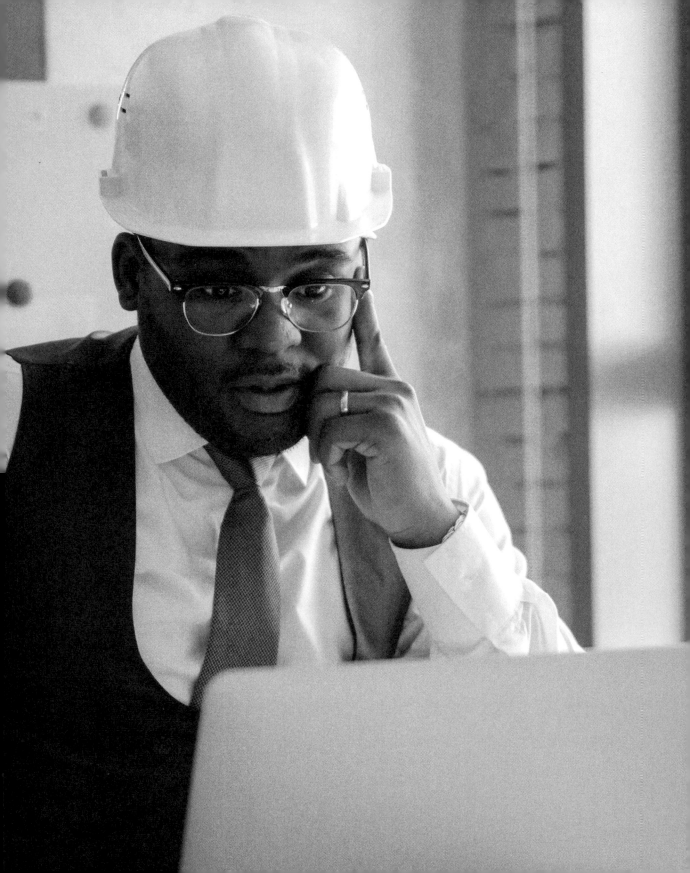

CHAPTER 10

Living well

You've lived through an unpleasant bout of back or neck pain, but you're feeling better and you're grateful to be back to your old routine. Now that the discomfort has subsided and your life is finally returning to normal, you no longer take your back and neck for granted. You want to know how to care for your body and avoid another painful episode in the future.

While there's no foolproof way to prevent another flare up, you can make choices every day to reduce the chances that pain will come knocking again at your door. Healthy-living choices, including exercise and activity, proper posture, and managing your weight, sleep and stress level, all play an important role in caring for your back and neck. By making these areas of life a priority, you'll have a better chance of staying pain-free.

EXERCISE AND PHYSICAL ACTIVITY

It's common knowledge that exercise is good for your health and well-being. Exercising strengthens your heart, boosts your mood, and helps prevent or manage many health problems and concerns. But did you know that exercise is good for your back and neck, too?

Exercise not only improves painful back and neck conditions but can help prevent new problems from occurring. People who exercise regularly and are physically active generally have less back and neck pain and recover faster from pain and injury than do those who are less active.

Regular exercise strengthens the muscles, joints and bones that support your back and neck. Some research suggests that exercises such as brisk walking and running may forti-fy the disks between the vertebrae by fueling them with blood and nutrients. Exercising can also help you achieve or maintain a healthy weight and lower stress, both of which reduce your risk of hurting your back and neck.

How much?

For most healthy adults, the U.S. Depart-ment of Health and Human Services recom-mends at least 150 minutes of moderate aer-obic activity or 75 minutes of vigorous aerobic activity weekly, or a combination of the two. Moderate activity, such as brisk walking, requires medium effort. It increas-es your heart rate and breathing, but you can still hold a conversation. Vigorous activ-ity, such as jogging or running, uses greater effort, making it difficult to say more than a couple of words without a breath.

Guidelines also recommend doing strength training exercises for all major muscle groups at least two times a week.

It's best to spread your exercise sessions throughout the week. You're more likely to injure your neck or back if you try to squeeze all your activities into one or two days. If possible, try to get at least 30 minutes of moderate physical activity most days of the week. If you don't have long chunks of available time, you can break up those 30 minutes throughout the day. For instance, if you can't fit in a 30-minute walk, try to do three 10-minute walks instead.

Getting started

If regular exercise is already part of your weekly routine, good for you. Keep at it. If you're like many people who haven't been physically active in a while, getting started might seem daunting. It doesn't have to be. The key is to start small, building your strength and endurance over weeks or months.

If you've been inactive for a long time or if you have a chronic health condition, make an appointment with your doctor first be-fore beginning an exercise program. Then think about the sorts of activities you enjoy doing. Maybe it's walking, dancing or go-ing to a yoga class with a friend.

If you're not sure what you like, give differ-ent types of exercise a try. Don't force your-self to keep doing something you don't en-joy. The best kind of exercise is the kind you're willing to do and will stick with.

Once you're ready to begin a new exercise routine, ease into it. If you do too much too soon, you could injure yourself or get dis-couraged. It's better to start slowly, gradual-ly increasing your effort and your intensity level as your fitness level improves.

Stretching and strengthening

As part of your exercise routine, be sure to include basic back and neck stretches most days of the week. Stretching is important because it helps loosen tight muscles and keeps your back and neck limber, lowering your risk of muscle strain and other injuries.

Also include exercises that strengthen your core — the muscles around your torso and pelvis — and your neck. Core and neck exercises help prevent problems by strengthening the muscles that support your spine.

Research suggests that a combination of basic stretches, strengthening exercises and aerobic activity can help prevent pain in people with back and neck conditions. You can find examples of stretching and strengthening exercises in Chapter 7.

Aerobic activity

In addition to stretching and strengthening exercises, you want to include aerobic activity in your exercise routine. Aerobic activity works large muscle groups, increases your heart rate and has many health benefits.

Regular aerobic activity reduces pain and promotes back and neck health by increasing blood flow to your muscles, improving flexibility, strengthening your core and improving your fitness. Aerobic exercise also improves the functioning of your heart and lungs and lowers your risk of diseases such as diabetes, heart disease and cancer.

Running, swimming, bicycling and active sports such as tennis are all types of aerobic activity. So are daily activities like gardening, housekeeping, taking the stairs and walking the dog. No particular type of aero-bic exercise is better than another when it comes to back and neck conditions. What matters is that you choose those activities you enjoy the most so that you stay active.

Walking If you're new to aerobic exercise or have been inactive for a while, walking is a good place to start. Walking is a safe, simple and low-impact aerobic activity that you can do just about anywhere.

Before you begin, be sure to choose comfortable clothing and a good pair of walking shoes. Your shoes should have proper arch support, a firm heel, and thick flexible soles that cushion your feet and absorb shock.

Remember, it's OK to start slowly — especially if you haven't been exercising regularly. You might begin with five minutes a day the first week, and then increase your time by five minutes each week until you reach at least 30 minutes.

During your walks, aim to move as fast as you're able. As your fitness level increases from week to week, you can gradually increase the pace of your walks. Brisk walks promote back health and reduce pain more than do leisurely strolls. Compared with a slow walk, walking briskly with your arms swinging at your sides allows for more spinal movement and places significantly less pressure on your back muscles and vertebrae. Brisk walks are also better for your overall health.

Water exercise Water (aquatic) exercise is another low-impact aerobic activity that can

WALK WELL

Your posture and technique are important when walking. To protect your spine and gain fitness benefits, follow these recommendations:

- **Head.** Hold your head level, with your chin parallel to the ground. Point your eyes forward, not down.
- **Shoulders and arms.** Move your shoulders and arms naturally as you walk, with your arms bent slightly at the elbow.
- **Back and neck.** Keep your back comfortably straight, with your spine in a neutral position. (See page 177 to find your neutral spine position.) Keep your body weight over the middle of your feet. Try not to lean forward on your toes or back on your heels.
- **Core.** Engage the core muscles of your back and abdomen by gently pulling your bellybutton toward your spine while breathing normally.
- **Feet.** Walk smoothly, rolling each foot from heel to toe.

be helpful if you have a back condition. The buoyancy of water supports your body weight and takes the pressure off your bones, joints and muscles. Water is also much harder to move through than is air, which means your body has to work harder. This natural resistance helps you strengthen your muscles — including your core — and improves your overall fitness. Exercising in warm water can also soothe pain, allowing you to move more freely.

You can do water exercise even if you don't know how to swim. Simply walking across a pool in waist-high water is good for your muscles and joints. You can also walk through deeper water by wearing a flota-tion belt that keeps you upright. If you're looking for more guidance or variety, try a water exercise class. Many fitness centers offer classes that are suitable for nonswimmers and swimmers alike.

Other helpful exercises

Along with traditional aerobic exercise, there are other low-impact activities you might find beneficial. These activities may also be a good place to start if you're struggling to commit to an exercise routine. While they may not satisfy all of your aerobic activity needs, the exercises can help you enjoy different types of physical activity.

Yoga Yoga is a mind-body practice that may help prevent or manage back or neck pain by reducing your stress level and tension in your muscles. It also helps improve strength, flexibility and balance. Yoga combines physical poses, controlled breathing, and meditation or relaxation. It also combines physical and mental disciplines with the intent of achieving peacefulness of body and mind.

Yoga has many styles, forms and intensities. Hatha is one of the most common styles of yoga, and beginners may like its slower pace and easier movements. But most people can benefit from any style of yoga; it's all about your personal preferences.

Although you can learn yoga from books and videos, beginners usually find it helpful to start with an instructor. Yoga studios offer classes, as do many fitness and community centers. Before starting a class, ask about the instructor's training and experience, and make sure the class is suitable for your experience level. Many people combine classes with yoga sessions at home. Some people practice yoga once or twice a week, while others do it more often.

Tai chi Tai chi is a graceful form of exercise that involves a series of movements performed in a slow, focused manner and accompanied by deep breathing. Often described as meditation in motion, tai chi promotes serenity through gentle, flowing movements.

When learned and practiced correctly, tai chi can help treat and manage back and neck problems by increasing strength, flexibility and balance and by reducing stress. Although you can use videos and books to learn how to do tai chi, consider seeking guidance from a qualified tai chi instructor to gain the activity's full benefits and learn proper techniques. You can find tai chi classes at many fitness centers, health clubs and community centers.

While you may benefit from a class that lasts 12 weeks or less, you may enjoy greater benefits if you continue tai chi for the long term and become more skilled. You also may find it helpful to practice tai chi at home every day to develop a routine.

Qi gong Closely related to tai chi, qi gong combines mindful breathing, meditation and slow, rhythmic movements. Qi gong is commonly performed standing, but some forms are done in sitting or lying positions. Qi gong can reduce stress and pain, and some research suggests that it may help people manage neck and back conditions.

If possible, begin with the guidance of an experienced instructor. To find a class near you, contact local fitness and community centers or the community education department of your local school district. If you can't find a class in your community, books and videos can teach you the basics of qi gong. To get the most benefit, try to practice qi gong daily.

Pilates Pilates is a form of exercise that consists of low-impact movements to increase flexibility, as well as muscular strength and endurance. Pilates can help you build strength in your core muscles, leading to better posture, stability and balance. For these reasons, Pilates may be beneficial for back and neck health.

A common misperception is that Pilates requires specialized equipment. Maybe you've seen a Pilates apparatus, called a reformer, that looks like a bed frame with a sliding carriage and adjustable springs. Don't let these machines intimidate you. Many Pilates exercises can be done on the floor with just a mat.

Because it's essential to maintain the correct form to gain the most benefit — and to avoid injuries — beginners should start out under the supervision of an experienced Pilates instructor. Be sure to let your instructor know about any ongoing or previous back or neck injuries so that he or she can assist you in modifying movements.

IMPROVING YOUR POSTURE

As you go about your day, your posture is probably the last thing on your mind. But the way you stand, sit and lift can make a big difference when it comes to your neck and your back.

With correct posture, your body is lined up and balanced so that all of your body structures are supported. Good posture also takes less energy to maintain than does poor posture. Poor posture can lead to weak, tight muscles and overstretched ligaments,

place additional stress on your spine, and increase your risk of neck and back pain. By paying a little extra attention to the way you stand, sit and lift, you'll be doing your back and neck a big favor.

Stand smart

Have you ever been told to stand straight or stop slouching? Good posture is about more than just the way you look. It can have a positive effect on your health, especially back and neck health. Use these tips to maintain a healthy posture while standing:

- **Head.** Hold your head level so that your chin is parallel to the floor and your head is balanced over your shoulders.
- **Shoulders.** Keep your shoulders relaxed and balanced over your hips.
- **Neck and back.** Keep your neck and back relaxed and comfortably straight. Avoid slouching.
- **Hips.** Maintain a healthy spine position (neutral spine) by making sure your pelvis isn't tilted too far forward or backward.
- **Core.** Engage your core muscles by gently pulling your bellybutton toward your spine. Keep this bracing position as you breathe normally.
- **Feet.** Stand with your toes pointed forward and your feet parallel to one another. Wear comfortable, low-heeled shoes.

Even with correct posture, try not to stand for long periods of time if possible. If standing is part of your job or daily routine, shift your weight frequently or rest one foot on a stool or small box from time to time.

FINDING YOUR NEUTRAL SPINE POSITION

The term *neutral spine* describes a healthy position where your back is correctly balanced. This balance gives you the greatest comfort and stability. Because no two bodies are exactly alike, your neutral spine position is unique to you. Keeping a neutral spine position while standing, sitting and moving helps protect your back and neck from injury. Take a moment to find your neutral spine position with one or more of these methods:

Lying down

Lie on your back on a flat surface with your hands on your hips. Slowly roll your hips so that they press against the surface. Then roll them forward to lift them away from the surface. Slowly move between these two positions to find your most comfortable position. This is your neutral spine position.

Sitting

Sit on the front half of a chair with your hands on your hips. Slowly roll your hips toward the back of the chair to sit up straight, arching your back, and pushing your chest outward. Then slowly roll your hips forward to round your back, moving your head and chest downward. Slowly move between these two positions. The most comfortable position for you is your neutral spine position.

Standing

Stand tall with your back close to a wall. With your hands on your hips, relax your shoulders, arms and knees. Slowly roll your hips backward to press your back toward the wall. Then slowly roll your hips forward to move your back away from the wall. Slowly move between these two positions to find your most comfortable position. This is your neutral spine position.

Sit smart

If you're like a lot of people, you spend hours each day sitting — whether at work, during your leisure time or both. Sitting for long periods of time can strain your back and neck, especially if your posture is poor. Use these tips to protect and support your body while sitting:

- **Head.** Hold your head level so that your chin is parallel to the floor and your head is balanced over your shoulders.
- **Shoulders.** Keep your shoulders relaxed, not elevated, rounded or pulled backward.
- **Neck and back.** Keep your neck and back comfortably straight. Avoid slouching.
- **Hips.** Maintain a healthy spine position (neutral spine) by making sure that your pelvis isn't tilted too far forward or backward.
- **Core.** Engage your core muscles by gently pulling your bellybutton toward your spine. Remember to breathe normally.
- **Knees.** Your knees should be bent at a right angle so they're level with your hips.
- **Feet.** Keep your feet flat on the floor, or on a footrest or block.

If your job or your lifestyle involves a lot of sitting, consider these additional tips:

- **Choose your chair wisely.** If possible, use a chair with good lower back support, a swivel base, and adjustable or removable armrests.
- **Position your chair to fit your height.** Raise or lower your chair so that both feet are flat on the floor. Your knees and hips should be bent at a right angle so that your knees are level with your hips. If your chair is too high and can't be lowered, consider using a footrest or block. If it's too low and can't be raised, find a different chair.
- **Position your armrests.** If your chair has adjustable armrests, lower them so that your elbows are near your waist and your shoulders can relax downward.
- **Provide added support.** Placing a pillow or rolled towel in the small of your lower back can maintain its normal curve.
- **Don't sit on your wallet.** If you normally keep your wallet in your back pocket, remove it before sitting (see page 101).
- **Give your knees space.** Adjust your seat so that it doesn't press into the back of your knees. Allow a gap of two to three finger widths between your chair and the back of your knees.
- **Take breaks.** Get up from your chair frequently to stretch or take a short walk.
- **Change positions.** Avoid sitting in the same position for too long. Shift your position throughout the time you're sitting.
- **Adjust your workspace.** Position your monitor or chair so that your eyes are level with the top of your screen. Keep your mouse and other frequently used tools within close range so that you're not reaching for them.

Lift smart

Whether you're picking up a crying toddler, lugging groceries to your door or moving heavy boxes at work, lifting is a part of life. It's also a major cause of back and neck pain.

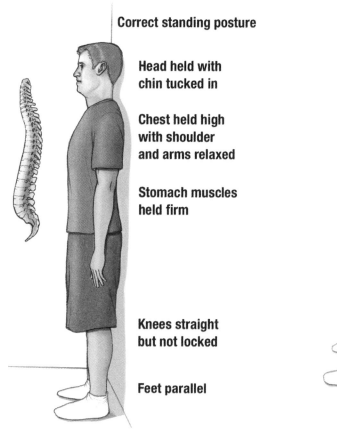

Correct standing posture

Head held with chin tucked in

Chest held high with shoulder and arms relaxed

Stomach muscles held firm

Knees straight but not locked

Feet parallel

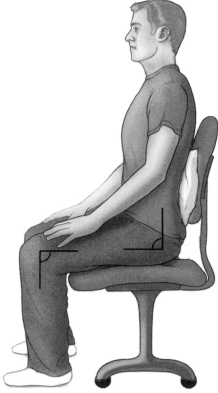

Correct sitting posture

Standing posture. Use the wall test to get a feel for good standing posture. Stand 2 to 4 inches from a wall and align your body as indicated above. Then walk away from the wall holding the proper posture.

Sitting posture. Keep your feet flat on the floor and maintain right angles at your knees and your hips. Your knees should be at the same height as your hips. Sit with your back straight and shoulders back yet relaxed.

While you may not be able to avoid lifting, you can help protect your body from injury by using proper lifting technique:

- **Consider alternatives.** Whenever possible, slide heavy objects rather than lift them. Or use a handcart or rollers to push the object.

- **Find a lifting partner.** Avoid lifting heavy objects on your own, especially if they weigh more than 50 pounds. If you do need to lift a heavy or awkward object, get one or more people to help you.

- **Plan.** Before moving a heavy object, decide where you'll place it and how to get it there.

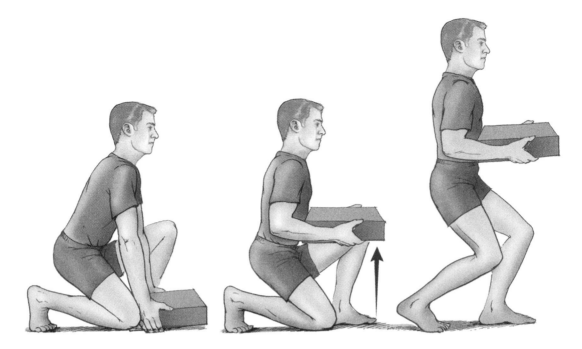

Proper lifting

Lifting posture. When lifting an object from the floor, first kneel next to the object. Next, lift the object onto your knee. Then, while maintaining the natural curves in your back, stand up, using your leg muscles to do the lifting.

- **Stand firm.** Plant your feet firmly on the ground before lifting. Make sure your body is centered over your feet. Stand as close to the object as possible.
- **Don't bend at the waist.** Let your legs do the work. Keeping your back straight -– no slouching — bend only at the knees. Once you have a firm grip on the object, use your leg muscles to rise to a standing position.
- **Hold the object close to you.** Carrying a load away from your body puts unnecessary strain on your spine.

- **Avoid twisting.** If you need to turn, pivot your feet so you aren't twisting at your waist.
- **Use your core muscles.** Pull your bellybutton toward your spine when lifting and carrying objects.
- **Center the object in front of you.** If possible, avoid carrying things on one side of your body. If you do, shift them from side to side periodically.

It might take a while to get used to correct standing, sitting and lifting practices, but keep at it. With time, these habits can become second nature. Also keep in mind that if you exercise regularly — maintaining your strength, stamina and flexibility — you don't have to worry as much about your posture and lifting mechanics. That's because individuals who are strong and fit tend to have better posture, and their spines are better suited for lifting.

If you continue to struggle with poor posture, talk to your doctor or consider working with a physical therapist.

IMPROVING YOUR WEIGHT

You may not realize it, but your weight can have a major effect on the health of your back and neck. People who are overweight are more likely to struggle with back or neck pain, in part due to the added pressure on the spine. Being at a healthy weight places less stress on your back and neck, which can help reduce and help prevent back and neck pain.

There's no doubt that achieving and maintaining a healthy weight can be challenging, but the extra effort is well worth it. If you're overweight, even a modest loss of weight may improve lower back pain significantly. A healthy weight comes with many other benefits, too, including improved heart health, increased energy levels and better self-esteem, to name a few.

What's a healthy weight?

Before launching into a weight-loss plan, first determine whether you need to lose weight. What's considered a healthy weight varies from person to person, but three factors can help you determine if you need to lose some weight.

Body mass index (BMI) Your BMI factors your height and weight in determining whether you have a healthy or unhealthy percentage of body fat. A BMI of 18.5 to 24.9 is considered a healthy range (see page 185). Keep in mind that BMI is a good but imperfect guide. Muscle weighs more than fat, for instance, so if you're very muscular and physically fit, you can have a high BMI without added health risks.

Waist circumference Waist circumference measures how much abdominal fat you have. Too much abdominal fat is linked to a greater risk of heart disease and other related conditions, such as high blood pressure, high cholesterol and diabetes. A measurement exceeding 40 inches in men and 35 inches in women is associated with increased health risks.

Medical history To get a more complete picture of your weight status, you might talk to your doctor. Along with your BMI and waist circumference, a thorough evaluation of your medical history can help determine if you need to lose some weight.

Setting SMART goals

If you've determined that now is a good time to start losing weight, you'll find no shortage of fad diets, weight-loss programs and outright scams promising you a quick and easy weight loss. Instead of navigating all of this

on your own, consider meeting with your doctor or a dietitian to discuss how to best go about losing weight successfully.

The foundation for any effective weight-loss plan is a commitment to making changes in your diet and exercise habits. Weight loss happens when you reduce extra calories from food and beverages, and increase calories burned through physical activity.

While that sounds simple, it can be difficult to put into practice. That's where SMART goals come in. SMART stands for specific, measurable, attainable, relevant and time-limited. It means starting off with small, reasonable goals and a concrete plan for how to achieve them.

- **Specific.** State exactly what you want to achieve, how you're going to do it, and when you want to achieve it. For example, instead of saying you'll exercise more, set a goal of walking 30 minutes after work every day. Instead of saying you'll improve your diet, aim to swap your afternoon sugary snack for a serving of fresh fruit.
- **Measurable.** Track your progress by measuring it. Wear a watch or activity device to monitor the length of your walks or workouts. Use an app or log to record the changes you're making to your diet. Recording your accomplishments can keep you motivated.
- **Attainable.** Set a goal that's realistic and that you can achieve with the time and resources you have available.
- **Relevant.** Set goals that are relevant and meaningful to you and that fit with

where you're at in your life right now. Don't set goals that someone else wants you to reach. Ask yourself what's most important to you.

- **Time-limited.** Pick a deadline for your goal that you can realistically meet. For example, if you want to work toward swimming 30 minutes twice a week, circle a date on the calendar to reach that goal and strive for that.

If you find that your goals are consistently too easy or hard, make adjustments as you go along. Be focused yet flexible.

GETTING ENOUGH SLEEP

When life gets busy, it can be tempting to skimp on sleep. But a good night's sleep is essential for your physical and mental health. A restful night allows your brain and body — including your back and neck — to recover from the day's activities, challenges and stresses. It prepares you for the next day and helps you to be your best.

Most adults need seven to nine hours of sleep a night to awaken feeling refreshed, alert and able to carry out their daily activities. Regularly getting less than seven hours of sleep isn't only hard on your back and neck but also can increase your risk of other health problems, such as weight gain, diabetes, heart disease, high blood pressure and stroke.

If sleep eludes you, try establishing consistent sleep habits. For example, stick to a reg-ular bedtime and follow a nightly pre-sleep ritual, such as a warm bath, muscle relaxation, gentle stretching or reading.

Your mattress and pillow

A supportive mattress and pillow are important for a good night's sleep. The right mattress for you is one that feels comfortable and supports the natural curves of your spine. It should allow you to wake up feeling rested and pain-free.

If you typically wake up in pain or feeling sore, you might consider purchasing a new mattress. A handful of small studies suggest that medium-firm mattresses or adjustable air-supported sleep systems may be better than firm mattresses. But more research is needed.

When it comes to your pillow, use one that keeps your neck in line with your chest and back. A pillow placed under your head should be high enough that it supports your neck's alignment but not so high that your neck is elevated above the rest of your body. Another option if you sleep on your back is to place a small pillow under the nape of your neck.

Sleep positions

Are you a back sleeper or a side sleeper? Or do you usually wind up on your stomach? Sleep position can either help or hinder back and neck health. Whatever your sleeping

WHAT'S YOUR BMI?

To determine your BMI, find your height in the left column of the table on the opposite page. Follow that row across to the weight nearest yours. Look at the top of that column for your approximate BMI. Or use this formula:

1. Multiply your height (in inches) by your height (in inches).
2. Divide your weight (in pounds) by the results of the first step.
3. Multiply that answer by 703. (For example, a 270-pound person, 68 inches tall, has a BMI of 41.)

My BMI :
_____

5'8" = 68"

① 68 × 68 = 4624

② $\frac{270}{4624}$ = 0.058391

③ 0.058391 × 703 = 41.048873

	Normal		Overweight					Obese				
BMI	**19**	**24**	**25**	**26**	**27**	**28**	**29**	**30**	**35**	**40**	**45**	**50**
Height	Weight in pounds											
4'10"	91	115	119	124	129	134	138	143	167	191	215	239
4'11"	94	119	124	128	133	138	143	148	173	198	222	247
5'0"	97	123	128	133	138	143	148	153	179	204	230	255
5'1"	100	127	132	137	143	148	153	158	185	211	238	264
5'2"	104	131	136	142	147	153	158	164	191	218	246	273
5'3"	107	135	141	146	152	158	163	169	197	225	254	282
5'4"	110	140	145	151	157	163	169	174	204	232	262	291
5'5"	114	144	150	156	162	168	174	180	210	240	270	300
5'6"	118	148	155	161	167	173	179	186	216	247	278	309
5'7"	121	153	159	166	172	178	185	191	223	255	287	319
5'8"	125	158	164	171	177	184	190	197	230	262	295	328
5'9"	128	162	169	176	182	189	196	203	236	270	304	338
5'10"	132	167	174	181	188	195	202	209	243	278	313	348
5'11"	136	172	179	186	193	200	208	215	250	286	322	358
6'0"	140	177	184	191	199	206	213	221	258	294	331	368
6'1"	144	182	189	197	204	212	219	227	265	302	340	378
6'2"	148	186	194	202	210	218	225	233	272	311	350	389
6'3"	152	192	200	208	216	224	232	240	279	319	359	399
6'4"	156	197	205	213	221	230	238	246	287	328	369	410

Based on *Circulation*, 2014;129(suppl 2):S102; NHBLI Obesity Expert Panel, 2013.

Asians with a BMI of 23 or higher may have an increased risk of health problems.

RELAXATION TECHNIQUES TO MANAGE STRESS

Learning how to relax in the face of stress takes practice. These techniques can help you calm your body and mind.

Relaxed breathing

Sit or lie in a comfortable position. Rest one hand comfortably on your abdomen and the other hand on your chest. Inhale slowly through your nose while pushing your abdomen out. Then slowly exhale through your mouth while pushing your abdomen in. Concentrate on breathing this way for a few minutes and become aware of the hand on your abdomen rising and falling with each breath. Make each breath a smooth, wavelike motion.

Progressive muscle relaxation

Sit or lie in a comfortable position, and close your eyes. Allow your jaw to drop and your eyelids to be relaxed but not tightly closed. Tighten the muscles in one area of your body and hold them for a count of five. Release the tightness completely and move on to the next part of your body. You may want to start by tensing and relaxing the muscles in your toes and progressively working your way up to your neck and head. You can also start with your head and neck and work down to your toes.

Guided imagery

Breathe slowly, regularly and deeply. Once you're more relaxed, imagine a calming place — somewhere you feel safe, happy and comfortable. Use all of your senses to notice every detail about this great place. What do you see, hear and smell? What do you feel with your hands and under your bare feet? After five or 10 minutes, rouse yourself gradually.

preferences, you can help support your spine with these small adjustments.

On your back When sleeping on your back, try placing a pillow under your knees. This can help straighten your spine and relax your back and neck muscles.

On your side If you're a side sleeper, drawing your knees up into a fetal position can help take pressure off your spine and open up space between your vertebrae. Another option is to bend one or both knees slightly and place a pillow between them. The pillow helps align your spine, pelvis and hips.

On your stomach This position can put stress on your back and neck, so it's better to avoid it if possible. But if you do sleep on your stomach, try placing a pillow under your stomach to relieve pressure from your spine.

LIMITING STRESS

The kids are screaming. The bills are due. The pile of papers on your desk is growing at an alarming pace. Stress is something that most people know well and experience often. It's a normal psychological and physical reaction to the demands of life. A small amount of stress can be good, motivating you to perform well. But too much stress can affect your overall health and well-being.

People's bodies respond to stress in different ways. Your friend might experience head-aches, stomachaches or jaw pain. For you, stress may produce muscle tension in your back and neck. This tension can contribute to back and neck problems. Left unchecked, stress can also suppress the body's immune system and increase the risk of other health problems, including heart and blood vessel disease.

Learning to recognize and manage stress can improve your health and help you care for your body. The next time your back or neck starts hurting, ask yourself if stress could be part of the problem. If the answer is yes, arm yourself with these stress-busting strategies.

- **Find ways to relax.** Techniques such as relaxed breathing, muscle relaxation, guided imagery and meditation can help ease muscle tension, lower your heart rate and clear your mind. Other stress-busters include watching a funny movie or taking a warm bath.
- **Simplify.** Break bigger projects into small tasks, focusing on one task at a time.
- **Prioritize.** Focus on what's important to you and set realistic goals. If you're over-committed, pare down the number of activities you're involved in, and say no to new commitments.
- **Get enough sleep.** Along with rejuvenating your body, sleep helps you tackle problems in a refreshed state.
- **Exercise.** Exercise releases brain chemicals that may leave you feeling happier, more relaxed and less anxious. It also helps burn off the excess energy and tension that stress can produce.

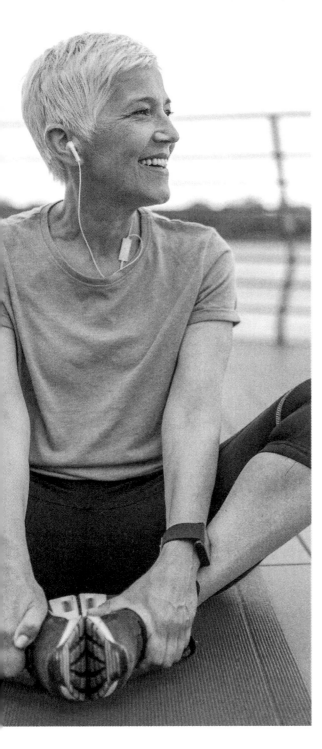

- **Eat well.** Enjoy healthy meals and snacks and limit caffeine. Too much caffeinated coffee, tea or soda will increase your stress level.
- **Do what you enjoy.** This may include going to the movies, joining a book club, hiking with friends or getting together for a game of cards. Doing something fun helps improve your mood and takes your mind off your worries.
- **Seek spirituality.** You may find spirituality in nature, art, music, meditation, prayer or by attending religious services. Nurturing your spirituality can help reduce stress by taking you outside yourself, giving you a greater sense of purpose and strengthening your connection to the world around you.
- **Talk to a trusted friend.** Talking can help relieve stress and put things in perspective, and it may lead to a healthy plan of action.
- **Develop a support network.** Family members, friends and co-workers whom you can turn to for emotional and practical support can be very important when coping with stress.
- **Seek help.** Contact your doctor or a mental health professional if stress is building or you're not functioning well.

THE BIG PICTURE

Back and neck conditions are common, but they don't have to be life altering. If you engage in healthy habits, you can manage whatever problem you're facing, as well as help prevent another bout of pain in the future. Healthy habits aren't a guarantee that you'll never experience back or neck pain again, but they do significantly reduce your chances, as well as provide many additional benefits for overall health and well-being.

Back and neck health involves daily practices, such as exercise and good posture, to keep your spine properly aligned and your muscles strong. Knowing when to seek medical help and following through with recommended treatment also is important. Finally, being good to your whole self — body and mind — will help you to stay well and remain active so that you can get the most out of life.

Index

Page references in italics indicate illustrations, and t *indicates a table.*

reactive, 43
rheumatoid, 65
risk factors for, 42
spinal, 43
X-rays for, 83
aspirin, 97, 165
autoimmune disorders, 65
axial burst fracture, 54

B

back and neck pain
aching, 32
activity-related, 32–33
acute, 30
age-related, ix, 27–28
anxiety-related, 29
burning, 32
causes of, ix–x, 28–29, 36 (*see also* pain, identifying cause of)
in the cervical spine (*see* neck problems, common)
chronic, 30–31
with difficulty walking, 32
duration of, ix, 30, 33, 36, 95
with fever, 33
generalized, 31, *31*
localized, 31, *31*
with loss of fine motor movement, 32
in the lumbar spine (*see* back problems, common)
nerve-related, 32
with numbness/tingling, 32–33
prevalence of, vi, ix, 27, 35, 59
radiating, *31,* 31–32
risk factors for, ix–x, 27–29
spread to arms or hands, 24
spread to legs or feet, 24
stabbing, 32

treatments for, xi, 95–101 (*see also* heat; ice; medication; physical therapy; steroids; surgery; *and specific conditions)*
weight-related, 28, 36
when to see a doctor, 33
See also back problems, common; neck problems, common
back belts, 100
backpacks, heavy, 101
back problems, common, 35–57
accidents and injuries, 54–55
back brace for, 55, 99–100
cauda equina syndrome (spinal cord compression), 41, 50–51, 153
degenerative disease, 35, 41–47, *44–46* (*see also* arthritis)
facet joint disease, 43–44, *44,* 66, 67
infections, 55–56
joint inflammation, 51–52, *52*
muscle-related, 36–39, *37,* 37–39
myofascial pain, 38–39
nerve-related, 47–51, *48–50,* 152
nonspecific low back pain, 35–36
overview of, 35–36
pinched nerve, 47–48, *48*
sacroiliitis, 51–52, *52*
scoliosis, 52–54, *53,* 162
spinal deformities, 52–54, *53*
spondylosis and spondylolisthesis, 46–47 (*see also* malalignment and instability)
sprains, 36–38, *37*
strained muscles, 36–38, *37*
synovial cyst, 45, *45*
trauma and fractures, 54–55
tumors, 56–57, 149
See also disks; osteoporosis; spinal stenosis

malalignment (spondylolisthesis) and instability, 69–71, *70,* 84
marijuana (cannabis), medical, 100–101
massage, 98–99
mattresses, 101, 183
medial branch blocks, 141
medical history, 104, 182
medication, 96–97, 143–146
    See also steroids
microdiskectomy, 154
MRI (magnetic resonance imaging), 85–87, *87*
multifidus muscle, 21, *21*
muscle relaxants, 144–145
muscles
    deconditioning after surgery, 167
    pain related to, 36–39, *37*
    progressive relaxation of, 186
    spinal, 20–23, *21,* 23
    weakness of, 32, 40, 64
myelography, 89–90, *90*
myofascial pain, 38–39, 62–63

N

naproxen, 96, 144, 165
neck pain. *See* back and neck pain
neck problems, common, 59–77
    arthritis, 64–65
    bone spurs, 65–66, *66*
    cervical dystonia (spasmodic torticollis), 61
    degenerative disease, 64–66, *66*
    disk conditions, *63,* 63–64
    facet joint disease, 66, *67*
    malalignment (spondylolisthesis) and instability, 69–71, *70*
    muscle spasm, 62
    myofascial pain syndrome, 62–63
    neck brace for, 73, 100
    nerve-related, 66–69, *68–69,* 152
    osteoporotic fracture, 71–72, *72*
    ruptured disk, *63,* 63–64
    spinal cord injuries, 73–77
    spinal stenosis, 68–69, *69,* 152
    sprains and strains, *60,* 60–61
    trauma and fractures, 71–77, *72*
    whiplash, 71
nerve damage after surgery, 167
nerve-related conditions, 47–51, *48–50,* 66–69, *68–69,* 152
nerves, spinal, 13, 17–19, *18,* 24
    See also sciatic nerve
nerve stimulation, *142,* 142–143
nerve studies, 91–92
nonprescription pain relievers, 96–97, 143
nonspecific low back pain, 35–36
nonsteroidal anti-inflammatory drugs (NSAIDs), 96, 144–146
nonsurgical interventions, 131–147
    acupuncture, 133–135
    chiropractic care, 131–133
    injections, 135–140, *136,* 138–140
    medication, 143–146
    nerve stimulation, *142,* 142–143
    radiofrequency ablation, *141,* 141–142
    traction, 143
nortriptyline, 145
NSAIDs (nonsteroidal anti-inflammatory drugs), 96, 144–146
nucleus pulposus, *16*
numbness/tingling, 32–33, 40, 64, 67

O

obesity. *See* overweight/obesity
oblique muscles, internal and external, 23

steroids
    for arthritis, 42
    for facet joint disease, 44
    injections of, 137
    for muscle pain, 37
    for pinched nerve, 48
    for a ruptured disk, 41, 64
    for sacroiliitis, 51–52
strains. *See* sprains and strains
stress, 29, 186–188
stretching, 97–98, 106–107, *109–115,* 172–73
superficial extrinsic muscles, 21
superficial intrinsic muscles, 20
surgery, 149–69
    anterior approach, 150, *150*
    bleeding (hematoma) after, 166
    bone removal, 153
    for bone spurs, 152
    for cauda equina syndrome, 51, 153
    for cervical myelopathy, 69
    complication risks of, 160
    corpectomy, 153
    decompression, 152–154, *154*
    deconditioning after, 167
    diskectomy, 153–154, 167
    disk herniation after, 167
    disk pain after, 167
    disk replacement, 162, *163,* 164
    elective, 149
    endoscopic diskectomy, 154
    facetectomy, 153
    facet replacement, 164
    failed back surgery syndrome (FBSS), 168–169
    foraminotomy, 153
    getting a second opinion, 157
    image-guided, 158
    infection after, 166–167
    joint pain after, 167

    laminectomy, 153, *154*
    laminoplasty, 153
    laminotomy, 153
    lateral approach, 151
    limitations after, 164–166
    malalignment and instability, 71
    microdiskectomy, 154
    minimally invasive, *151,* 151–153
    motion preservation, 162, *163,* 164
    nerve damage after, 167
    open, 151, *151,* 153
    outpatient, 152
    pain after, ongoing, 166–168
    for pinched nerve, 48, 149
    posterior approach, *150,* 150–151
    and preexisting conditions, 167–168
    pseudarthrosis after, 167
    as rarely necessary, vi, 36, 149
    robot-guided, 158
    for a ruptured disk, 41, 152
    for scoliosis, 54, 162
    for spinal deformities, 149, 161–162
    for spinal fractures, 54–55
    spinal fusion (stabilization), 154–156, 158, *159,* 160–62
    for spinal infection, 56
    spinal instability after, 167
    spinal stenosis after, 167
    for a synovial cyst, 45
    for tumors, 149, 161
Swedish massage, 99
synovial cyst, 45, *45*
synovium, 17, *17*

T

tai chi, 175
tailbone (coccyx), *15,* 16
tendons, 20, 36

IMAGE CREDITS

The individuals pictured are models, and the photos are used for illustrative purposes only. There is no correlation between the individuals portrayed and the subjects being discussed.

All photographs and illustrations are copyright of MFMER, except for the following:

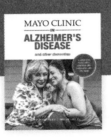
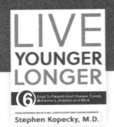
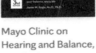
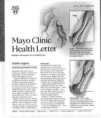